Weight Control with Asian Foods

Kay Shimizu

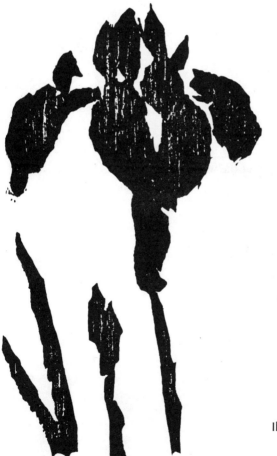

Illustrations by
Lois Shimizu

© Copyright in Japan 1975 by Kay Shimizu
Illustrations by Lois Shimizu
First Printing 1975

Published by Shufunotomo Co., Ltd.
1-chome, Surugadai, Kanda, Chiyoda-ku, Tokyo, 101 Japan

Exclusive Distributor in U.S.A. & Canada:
JAPAN PUBLICATIONS TRADING CO. (U.S.A.), INC.
• 200 Clearbrook Road, Elmsford, N.Y. 10523, U.S.A.
• 1255 Howard St., San Francisco, Calif. 94103, U.S.A.
ISBN: 0-87040-355-9

Printed in Japan

Introduction

Dear Friend: This is entirely a new kind of book—no counting of calories and at the same time presenting you a treasure-filled volume of easy to prepare Asian style recipes. I do not intend to make for an unhappy experience in your "often dieting" life. It is to encourage you to begin a habit of using practically "made to order diet" Asian foods to achieve your desired weight and to keep it under control.

Basically, Asian style is diet oriented and relatively less fattening ingredients are used. One's body has needs for a certain amount of unsaturated fats for a rounded out diet otherwise tolerance of all foods becomes so very touchy you could never eat and enjoy a meal. I do not mean weight control to achieve skinny bodies only. I am of the school which believes every person is happiest with a different weight ideal. Be comfortable and presentable. Do not risk poor health.

Naturally, every new flavor may not appeal to you from the very outset. Some flavors have to grow on you. Good Asian style foods are simple to prepare. This book features tempting dishes—imaginative taste-tested ideas for the "same old basics." These are recipes which have been developed with authentic ingredients but adapted to the tastes of Westerners without sacrifice of good flavors—some are definitely Chinese or Japanese and others are a combination of the best of each to yield good results.

Categories have been set up to make serving and selecting a menu simpler for you. Most of the recipes are relatively low in fats, salt and other factors that would make one tend toward heaviness. I am American with a good background luckily in Asian culture and life. I know how it is with a household especially the children who love hamburgers, hot dogs, chili, etc. Having taught Asian cooking to thousands in California I can know first hand the pulse of the American family and what they really like to eat in the average home.

This book is for families, for cooks and for gourmets. Most of us like

5

to think that we are fantastic cooks or we wouldn't continually be trying out new ideas. We want basically to be happy while we cook and this leads to the most important feature about cooking. If you cook with an attitude of enthusiasm, love and care your result will be so much better than if you cook with disgust and a feeling that here we are doing this same old boring "job" again.

I have tested this theory on myself and discovered it to be so true. Your vibrant spirit, your bubbling excitement and anticipation will insure success. Your ultimate reward will be the discovery that you have mastered the dish to your taste satisfaction.

Feel free to pick and combine dishes to make up your own menu. There is no need to make everything Chinese or all Japanese. Choose a recipe from one country and another dish from your Western cookbook. Use ingenuity and be creative!

The main point to remember is that you must balance your diet daily so that you will not be serving only meat or only one vegetable, etc. Our basic needs for body building daily continue throughout life. It is most urgently vital that you follow a good regimen of vitamin and mineral intake and be calorie-wise.

I have honestly tried to be nutritionally sound and suggest that you give serious thought to the amount you consume. Stick to about ½ cup of cooked rice which by the way symbolizes long life and fertility. You will find that it is only 100 calories and if you can "nurse" that one bowl throughout your meal you can concentrate upon your low calorie entrée.

Effective careful use of the test selected recipes in this book should result in good vibrant health with the added bonus of moderate weight because the fat developing factors just are not in the menus. Occasionally you can "cheat" without disastrous results.

You can even use lecithin spray (comes in a pressurized can) to coat your frying pan if you wish to further reduce your usage of oils. But do it cautiously. Even an ingredient like sugar is only 16 calories per teaspoon so when a little is used in the recipe and it is divided among many persons it is not much. Far less than drinking down one bottle of sodapop or a cocktail which both contain many empty calories.

To be overweight brings excessive burden for your heart, your joints and your entire physical being as well as affecting your mental attitudes.

I wish you good cooking, fine feasting and above all a loss or a gain in weight as the case may be. Enjoy!

Cordially yours,
Kay Shimizu
Saratoga, Ca.

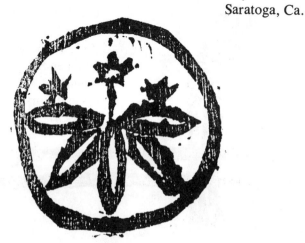

CONTENTS

Measurement Conversion
1 cup = 240 c.c. = 8 ounces
1 Tablespoon = 3 teaspoons
1 pound = 454 grams
1 Tablespoon = 15 c.c.
1 teaspoon = 5 c.c.

Basic Rules

Even Asian style cooking requires moderation in eating. It is the key in any cuisine. Eating less of everything will help you to lose weight. And maintain control of yourself.

● Adjust the serving portion to meet your special needs. If you do however intend to become a *sumo* wrestler then by all means gorge yourself with rice, pans and pans of Asian style foods and you will surely become a big specimen!

● Avoid snacking or at least choose those foods low in calories.

● Zest and flavor can improve our meals especially if they are non caloric.

● Eat slowly and chew. This way you can relish the delightful flavors, the varied textures, the tantalizing aroma and benefit from the nutritive values. And above all gain less weight. You will feel satisfied as your desire for seconds will be curved. Hopefully, that is!

● Do not deprive yourself of certain foods because they are rich and fatty. These foods can be consumed but your portions should be very, very small. We could never be "that" rigid with our small indulgences.

● Tea has no calories unless you add sugar and cream. So learn to enjoy it in true Asian manner—no sugar. You will learn the real flavor and there are so many exquisite fragrances and endless varieties for you to experiment with. Usually with good tea the second infusion (the second pouring in of hot water over the tea leaves) is better than the first. I usually do not follow the instructions on the tea packages. I use tea leaves much more sparingly and my students and friends have enjoyed the delicate aroma even more.

● Carefully use flour, cornstarch, sugar, honey and other sweets. Use less salt and soy sauce. It will help reduce your retention of water which adds to weight. Regular eating habits tend to prevent fatigue or a desire to nibble at snacks and lessen our tendency to overeat in haphazard manner. Get plenty of sleep and rest.

● Losing weight gradually is more lasting. You will be happier mentally and your stomach will benefit from regularity!

● Choosing low calorie type foods: Thin, delicate, clear, fresh, watery or crisp are the watch words. High calorie foods are usually thick, oily, greasy-crisp, smooth, gooey, sweet and sticky, compact or concentrated, alcoholic. Use minimum quantities of fats, oils and sugar. Learn to experiment with the fascinating variety of condiments for seasonings. Often this will allow you to use less sauces and gravies which is good. Remove any visible and excess fat or skin on meat and poultry.

● You will in time develop a sort of intuition that will tell you the amount and the kinds of foods you can enjoy and still maintain proper weight control.

● Weighing regularly before breakfast once a week is a good idea. Always at the same time on the same day of the week. Do it consistently for awhile. Eventually you will not have to resort to your scale any more. We all know that there are some of us who feel best a little bit heavier than the fashion models and yet there are those thin persons who just drag when they are even a few pounds heavier. It is definitely an individual matter and I am the last one who would tell you that there is an ideal desirable weight for all persons.

● For uniform cooking time, for a beautiful appearance and

harmony as you cook try to cut meat and vegetables about the same size. Diagonal cutting style, cubes, dicing, mincing are all manners of the Chinese style.

● Japanese style differs somewhat and they give less attention to the uniformity of size and shape. Their emphasis is more on the natural aesthetic beauty of the vegetables served in season, arranged in decorative manner and cut with care. The visual portion of the food is most important. Many Japanese foods are prepared ahead and served at room temperature.

● We live in this modern age and do not depend upon traditional native ways although please stop often to appreciate the wonderful background that these ancient cultures offer. Ours is an entirely different life so very dependent upon the speedy pace of jet-age living. We have to harmonize new ideas with the changing times. Always think of today and have a great faith in the abundant joy of the future ahead. You will achieve your goal of weight control that way.

● And lastly my other books on the market will help you to learn more and more about Asian cooking. See the back cover for the listing. Good luck!

Appetizers, Salads and Potpourri

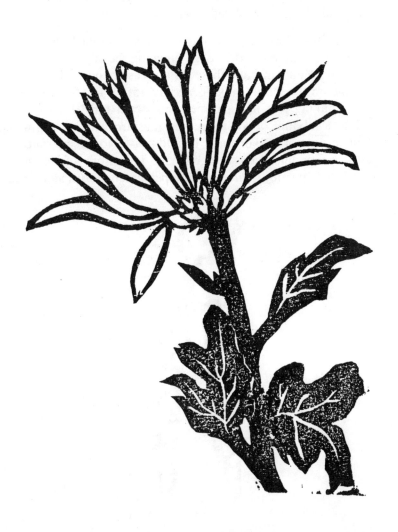

Lop Cheong in Wraps *(Chinese)*

Oven   *Serves many*

A quick and easy method of preparing an *hors d'oeuvre* and yet with authentic flavorings.

> ⅓ **pound Chinese sausages *(lop cheong)*, steamed for 15 minutes, then cut into ¾ inch pieces**
> **2 tubes of refrigerated biscuits or prepare your own favorite biscuit dough with 2 cups flour**

Remove ready-to-bake biscuits from container. Cut each one in half. Wrap around the cold cooked sausage pinching the edges of the dough together firmly. You can bake these on a greased cooky sheet for the specified time on the biscuit tube (generally 450°F for 10 minutes) or else place a baking pan in a steamer and steam for 10–15 minutes. Dipping into a mixture of soy sauce and mustard while eating makes the "tid-bit" even more flavorsome. To add "dash" to the dip sauce you could add one or all of these together: a few drops of sesame oil, chopped Chinese parsley *(cilantro)*, chopped green onions and vinegar.

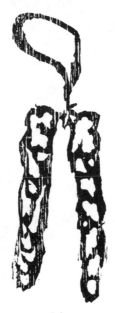

14

Chinese Pot Roast

Top of stove *Serves many*

Usually this is served cold on an appetizer plate. But nothing is stopping you from serving it hot if desired or using it as sandwich meat.

> **3 or 4 pound rump roast, boneless without much fat, cut in half**
> **1 cup light soy sauce (*shoyu*)**
> **2 or 3 Tablespoons sugar**
> **2 stalks green onion, tied in a knot**
> **a piece of fresh ginger root, 2 inches square**
> **¾ teaspoon Chinese 5-spice powder**
> **3 Tablespoons sherry wine**

Put all ingredients into a small but deep pot with a cover and allow to marinate for two hours if possible. Then place over high heat and bring to a boil. Lower heat and simmer for 1½ hours or until tender. Place meat on a dish to cool. Chill if time permits. This will allow the meat to firm up nicely and slicing it will definitely be simplified.

An electric knife will do a superb job of making even slices for your *hors d'oeuvre* tray. Garnish with Chinese parsley.

The flavored stock left over from cooking this meat can be saved and used over and over again for cooking meat, poultry or eggs. Each time slightly parboil the meat or whatever you plan to use to sterilize it before submerging in the flavored stock for further cooking. Add no vegetables. Keep in refrigerator during the storage period of any left-over stock. Be sure to boil it periodically so that bacterial action will not begin.

See recipe page 35 which uses this same flavored stock.

Spinach Relish *(Chinese)*

Top of stove   *Serves 4*

An entirely different approach to plain cooked spinach greens. Tasty, low calorie and yet highly nutritious. This dish goes well with almost any meal.

> **1 large bunch fresh spinach, washed well in slightly warm water to loosen sand, grit, etc. Since it is so difficult to decide sometimes as to the size of the bunch make enough to yield about ¾ cup cold, cooked spinach**
> **Ingredients A:**
> **1 teaspoon sesame oil, or more if desired**
> **1 teaspoon light soy sauce** *(shoyu)*
> **½ teaspoon sugar**
> **¼ teaspoon rice wine vinegar**
> **dash MSG (optional)**

Blanch spinach in plenty of boiling water for 1 minute. Drain and rinse in cold water. Drain carefully to remove all traces of water. Mince spinach. Mix ingredients A together with spinach in a bowl.

Chill in refrigerator. Serve this spinach as a side dish when serving a hot entrée.

A small rib of raw celery, 4 inches long, chopped fine, added to spinach just before mixing gives a very interesting texture to this relish.

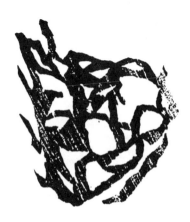

Fluffy Cellophane Salad *(Chinese)*

No cooking except blanching vegetable *Serves 4*

A most nutritional combination of exotic ingredients in this unusual salad. Healthy and yet non-fattening.

½ pound mung bean sprouts, washed and drained
1 ounce of agar-agar, string type or substitute *kanten*,
Japanese agar-agar (4 sticks equal 1 ounce)
3 ribs celery, shredded into matchstick lengths
1 cup cooked ham, shredded into matchstick lengths
3 green onions, cut like matchstick lengths, slivered

Put agar-agar in a bowl of cold water for about 20 minutes. Squeeze water through agar-agar with hands. This softens agar-agar (but does not melt it) and at the same time allows any sediment particles to loosen. Rinse several times more with cold water. Squeeze all excess moisture from agar-agar. Cut into shreds with a sharp cleaver.

Blanch mung bean sprouts with boiling water for 1 minute over high heat. Drain immediately and pour cold water to stop the cooking process. This will be just enough to remove the "raw" taste from the sprouts. Drain well. Mix all above ingredients together in a salad bowl and keep chilled until ready to be mixed with ingredients below.

2 teaspoons sesame oil
1 Tablespoon oil
1 Tablespoon rice wine vinegar
2 teaspoons soy sauce *(shoyu)*
1 teaspoon salt
½ teaspoon dry mustard
¼ teaspoon Chinese 5-spice powder

Toss gently just before serving to retain best flavors.

Intriguing Radishes *(Chinese)*

No cooking   *Serves many*

An exciting addition to any meal for an appetite whetting experience. Sweet and yet sour flavors.

> **1 large bunch red radishes having fresh appearing leaves,**
>   **wash well and cut off radishes from stems, saving leaves**
> **1 teaspoon salt**
> **Ingredients A:**
>   **1 teaspoon sesame oil**
>   **1½ teaspoons sugar**
>   **1 teaspoon soy sauce *(shoyu)***
>   **1½ Tablespoons rice wine vinegar**
>   **dash MSG (optional)**

Carefully smack the flat side of a heavy cleaver on radishes to crush. Not too hard!

Be careful not to break into pieces. Cut leaves into ¾ inch pieces. Sprinkle salt over all and mix. Allow to stand for about 10 minutes. Drain. Squeeze out excess juices. Mix ingredients A over the salted radishes. Toss to distribute flavors.

Serve cold as a sort of pickle relish.

Fresh Soy Beans *(Japanese)*

Top of stove   *Serves many*

Cooked fresh soy beans in the pod are a very Japanese way of serving this fantastic vegetable. Immature soy beans generally about 100 days after being planted are boiled whole in water with a dash of salt.

The pods are served usually at room temperature. Place the pod in mouth between the teeth and pull through slowly. The beans will pop out along with portions of the soft green pod.

Soy beans can be planted in the same manner that snap beans are grown. Seeds are planted in spring and the beans are picked when young and tender. Cooked as a vegetable soy beans add a new flavor to the diet.

For Westerners soy beans are the newest and most exciting addition to our daily diets but for centuries the nutritional value was known to the Asians. This is a most versatile and yet low calorie food. And practically all protein.

A substitute for this recipe could be fresh peas in the pod. Boil them as they come from the store—whole unshelled pods—ever so briefly and serve whole. They do not have to be served hot. They are fine served cold with beer or with dinner. The problem might be that one cannot find fresh peas in pods since so much of the crops are now sold as frozen products.

Cabbage Pickles *(Japanese)*

Toast seeds otherwise no cooking   *Serves many*

Like cole slaw but far less calories! This versatile tangy "salad" can be adapted to accompany any international meal.

1 pound round head of cabbage, shredded fine
1 small carrot, shredded fine
1 teaspoon salt
1 Tablespoon sugar
⅓ cup rice wine vinegar
2 Tablespoons white sesame seeds, toasted and partially
   crushed

Sprinkle salt on vegetables. Mix well. Add balance of ingredients. Mix again. Let this stand for about 1 hour before serving.

How to toast sesame seeds: Heat a dry heavy-weight frying pan over medium heat. Use no oil. Put in sesame seeds and keep shaking pan as seeds slowly become toasted and tan colored. Remove from pan and crush slightly using a Japanese *suribachi* or mortar and pestle. Another method to crush seeds: use a rolling pin over a sheet of waxed paper placed on top of toasted seeds.

Fruit Blossoms

Top of stove *Serves many*

Litchees are often called nuts but in reality the fresh delicious fruit has a pinkish brittle thin shell and sort of looks like a strawberry. The juicy litchee inside is pearly white. In America generally we must be satisfied with canned litchees but occasionally we can buy fresh ones. When this luscious fruit is dried it appears brownish. It can be compared with a raisin which starts out as a grape so succulent and as a raisin, dehydrated, its character changes to one of chewiness.

½ **pound fresh crab meat, cartilages removed, flaked**
1 **small can water chestnuts, finely chopped**
¼ **teaspoon salt**
1 **Tablespoon oil**
1 **10-ounce can litchees, drained (24 litchees), save liquid for other uses such as gelatin desserts, etc.**
Sauce ingredients:
1 **teaspoon curry powder**
1 **cup chicken broth**
1 **Tablespoon cornstarch**
dash MSG (optional)

Mix crab meat, water chestnuts and salt. Heat skillet on high heat. Add oil. Slosh around. Toss-fry about 2 minutes to blend flavors. Remove and cool.

Put a spoonful of this loose mixture into the litchee fruit cavity (where seed once lodged) which has been spread open. Place in shallow serving platter. Heat sauce ingredients in a small saucepan. Stir and cook until thickened. Pour hot sauce over your litchee "blossoms". Serve.

Any left-over filling can be piled under the "blossoms" or used in combination with cream cheese and worcestershire sauce for canapés.

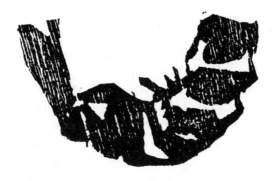

Hoisin Shrimp *(Chinese)*

Top of stove

Serves many
Serves 3 as entrée

Unexcelled for appetizers as well as a quick and simple main entrée for dinner. Add a vegetable dish, a light salad and your cosmopolitan meal is ready.

1 Tablespoon oil
1 clove garlic, minced
½ teaspoon fresh ginger root, grated
1 pound shrimp, shelled, deveined and washed
2 green onions, chopped
Ingredients A:
    2 teaspoons light soy sauce *(shoyu)*
    1 Tablespoon sherry wine
    2 Tablespoons *hoisin* sauce
    dash MSG (optional)

Heat skillet or wok. Add oil, garlic and ginger. Toss-fry ½ minute. Add shrimp and green onions toss-frying for 2 minutes. Add ingredients A. Stir until shrimp is rather dry and coated with flavorings. Should take about 3 minutes. Serve these attractively arranged on a contrasting colored platter for a good effect.

Salad of the Oceans *(Japanese)*

No cooking   *Serves 4*

Here is a delicacy from the ocean harvest which we truly should appreciate. My students who are often "first time tasters" love this concoction if they just don't think "seaweed". Westerners are not conditioned to seaweed as an edible plant as the Asians are. Slowly however with the advent of the health food craze more and more persons are becoming acquainted with this most nutritious product of the ocean....a sea vegetable.

> **1 cup canned shrimp, crabmeat, abalone or fresh seafood—even cooked octopus, sliced, is good**
> **A small handful of Japanese sliced dried seaweed *(wakame)* about 7–8 inches long to equal about 1 cup when soaked in water. This is most difficult to estimate—about 1¼ ounces in the dry state.**
> **1 large rib of celery or ½ of a large cucumber**
> **thin omelet made with 2 eggs**

Shred crabmeat (or leave small fresh local shrimps whole or jullienne strip canned abalone). Jullienne strip celery or the cucumber. Soak *wakame* in cold water to cover until soft—takes about 10 to 15 minutes. Rinse well to remove sand. Drain. Cut into 1 inch lengths. Make a very thin omelet using slightly beaten egg diluted with a bit of water or stock. Fry in lightly oiled frying pan at medium temperature until set. Let cool and cut into short strips (¼ × 1 inch). Mix all ingredients in bowl. Add following dressing:

> **6 Tablespoons rice wine vinegar**
> **2 Tablespoons sugar**
> **1 Tablespoon water**
> **½ teaspoon salt and ½ teaspoon soy sauce *(shoyu)***
> **1 teaspoon fresh ginger root, grated**
> **dash msg (optional)**

The above is a low calorie dressing for any green salad. The rice vinegar gives a most delicate flavoring and fragrance that is unsurpassed. Try it even for your home mixed salad dressings Western style.

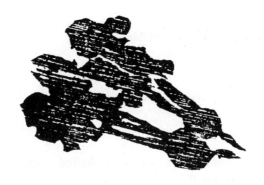

Chicken Soup *(Japanese)*

Top of stove   *Serves 4*

Japanese soups are simple to prepare and yet with imagination they can add much variation to your menus.

> **6 cups prepared Japanese soup stock *(dashi)*. Make this from concentrated Japanese soup base either powdered or liquid type.**
> **1 cup chicken breast meat, sliced 1 inch long thin strips**
> **salt to taste**
> **1 Tablespoon soy sauce *(shoyu)***
> **dash MSG (optional)**
> **2 teaspoons fresh ginger root, grated**
> **2 green onions, slivered in 1 inch lengths**
> **a few slices of lemon peel, ¾ × ¹⁄₁₆ inch wide**

Prepare soup stock. Heat. Add chicken strips and simmer about 5 minutes. If there is any fat or scum on surface skim off with a ladle. Add salt, soy sauce, wine and MSG. Stir to blend. Taste and adjust seasonings if desired.

Ladle soup into bowls. Garnish with a few green onions, bits of ginger and a strip of lemon peel.

Variation: Very tiny cubes of soy bean cake *(tofu)* could be added to this soup. But only a few pieces in each bowl. It is this very aesthetic application of artistry even with foods that makes Japanese cuisine a feast for the eyes.

Curried Shrimp *(Chinese)*

Top of stove

Serves 3 as entrée
Serves more as appetizer

Zesty flavored succulent shrimp which will bring many compliments to you.

> 1 **pound raw shrimp, shelled, deveined, washed and drained**
> 1½ **teaspoons curry powder (or more)**
> ¼ **teaspoon salt**
> ¼ **teaspoon sugar**
> **dash** MSG **(optional)**
> ½ **cup stock**
> 1 **Tablespoon oil**
> 3 **green onions, minced fine**

Heat pan. Add oil. Slosh around. Add shrimp, curry powder, sugar, salt and MSG (optional).

Stir-fry until well blended. Add stock and simmer 4 minutes. Sprinkle with green onions. This can be used as an entrée appetizer.

If shrimp are fairly clean veined you can skip deveining and leave shells intact. And proceed with recipe. Serve shrimp—shells and all. However discard shells as you eat!

Miso Dressing *(Japanese)*

No Cooking

Serves 2

This can be used for salads or for dips. *Miso* is a nondescript brown paste that is made from soy beans, rice and malt. It keeps indefinitely in the refrigerator and is a good source of minerals, vitamins and protein.

There are all kinds on the store shelf. Flavors and colors vary. But for the uninitiated I recommend buying the lightest one possible called *shiro miso* or literally translated white *miso* (appearance however is beige). It is somewhat sweet and lightly salted.

2 Tablespoons light *shiro miso*
1 teaspoon sugar
⅛ teaspoon dry mustard
1 Tablespoon rice wine vinegar/1 Tablespoon water
dash MSG **(optional)**

Stir all ingredients together until *miso* is well blended and the sugar is dissolved. Pour over your choice of raw or parboiled vegetables. It is also a good base for a dip with raw vegetables julienne cut.

Eggplant with Mustard Sauce *(Japanese)*

No cooking   *Serves many*

This is a firey-hot approach to using bland flavored eggplant which for some persons is a most tasteless vegetable. This "pickle" is quick and simple to prepare and can be made ahead.

> **2 or 3 medium-sized Japanese eggplant (elongated, slightly crescent shaped and midget compared to Black Beauty variety in United States). Use enough to make 1 ½ cups by measure. If Japanese variety is not available substitute a very tiny "large" Western type eggplant.**
> **about ½ teaspoon salt**
> **Ingredients A:**
> > **1 Tablespoon rice wine vinegar**
> > **1 Tablespoon sugar**
> > **1 Tablespoon soy sauce** *(shoyu)*
> > **1 Tablespoon dry mustard**

Put chopped eggplant in a bowl. Sprinkle with salt. Mix well with hands. Place a small saucer on top of eggplant. Put a heavy weight on top of saucer. After about 2 or 3 hours much of the water in the eggplant will be released. Squeeze eggplant firmly in palm of hands so all water is removed.

Make a sauce with ingredients A and mix with eggplant. Allow this to set about ½ day for best taste although in an emergency you could serve it immediately.

Delicate Fish Soup *(Japanese)*

Top of stove   *Serves 4*

Gourmets will glorify this humble soup as a favorite. Do not overly add the sauce—just enough to give you a delicate taste. This will be the charming part of this easily prepared soup. Very lean at that!

> **1 pound fish fillets (sea bass or red snapper), cut into 1 ×**
>   **½ inch pieces, salted lightly and allowed to set about 1**
>   **hour prior to use**
> **4 cups boiling water**
> **1 piece of *dashi konbu* (seaweed), 5 inches square**
> **1 block Japanese style soy bean cake *(tofu)*, cut into ½ ×**
>   **1 × ½ inch pieces**

Wash *konbu*. Place in bottom of large pan. Pour water and bring back to boiling point. Add salted fish pieces, carefully placing on *konbu*. Turn heat to very low and add *tofu*. Simmer just long enough to heat bean cake. Serve immediately with the following sauce and garnishes:

> **Mix together:**
>   **1 Tablespoon lemon juice**
>   **dash MSG (optional)**
>   **3 Tablespoons soy sauce *(shoyu)***
> **Garnishes:**
>   **1 green onion, chopped fine**
>   **½ cup fresh *daikon* root (Japanese white radish), grated**
>   **(This type of grating requires almost a puréed result.**
>   **Very easy to do in your blender)**

Usually the *konbu* is discarded but it still has many vitamins and nutrients and can be flavored with soy sauce *(shoyu)* and sugar to taste, cooked a brief period, cooled and cut into small pieces for snacking at another time.

Cream of Miso Soup *(Japanese)*

Top of stove   *Serves 4*

This is a traditional soup served quite regularly in Japan—probably most of the time, however, with a fish and seaweed base. This recipe substitutes chicken broth which is not quite so strongly flavored.

1 cup chicken broth
4 cups water
8 Tablespoons soy bean paste (*miso***—either white or red**
    types depending upon pungency desired—use white
    until you become accustomed to flavor since red types
    are saltier and more pronounced in taste)
dash MSG(optional)
2 green onions, chopped
1 cup Chinese cabbage*(nappa)***, sliced in thin strips**

Heat broth and water. When this boils add *miso*. Blend lumpy *miso* carefully into liquid. Lower heat. Add Chinese cabbage. Simmer 3 minutes. Add green onions. Cook ½ minute more. Serve immediately.

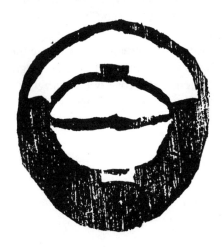

Edible Chrysanthemum Leaves *(Japanese)*

Top of stove   *Serves 4*

I always get strange looks when in class I tell my students that we are going to have chrysanthemum leaves today. This is a special variety and used frequently by the Japanese and the Chinese in their cuisine. The leaves are very tender and have a special taste which at first may not be very appealing to you. Again it is something that one acquires a taste for over a period of time.

> **1 large bunch *shungiku* (edible chrysanthemum), washed and drained**
> **Sauce ingredients:**
> > **1 Tablespoon soy sauce *(shoyu)***
> > **½ teaspoon sugar**
> > **1 Tablespoon sesame seeds, toasted and partially crushed**
> > **2 Tablespoons soup stock (Japanese *dashi* or full strength chicken stock can be used)**
> > **dash MSG (optional)**

Parboil *shungiku* about 2 minutes in lots of boiling water. Rinse and drain under cold water to cut the cooking process. The color should be very intense green.

Squeeze excess water from greens and arrange them in a neat straight line on your cutting board. Cut into 1½ inch lengths.

Mix sauce ingredients and toss with *shungiku* in a small bowl to blend flavors. Serve at room temperature.

Chicken with Horseradish *(Japanese)*

Top of stove   *Serves 4*

A very simple-to-prepare sophisticated appetizer. Uses *wasabi* powder (Japanese horseradish) which is a greenish tinge and very potent but most delightful in flavor. Some of my ambitious students use *wasabi* for their roast beef and sour cream accompaniment in place of regular white horseradish. In fact it grows on you! And its pungency certainly clears your sinuses.

1 cup chicken meat, cut from breast in thin slices 1 inch long
pot of boiling water
1 cup cucumber, cut like matchsticks
2 Tablespoons rice wine vinegar
dashes salt and MSG (optional)
1 teaspoon *wasabi* (Japanese green horseradish powder)
dashes light soy sauce *(shoyu)*
dash sugar
½ sheet of laver seaweed *(nori)*, toasted briefly holding over heat of stove, crushed with hands

Dip chicken slices for only a few seconds in boiling water using a slotted spoon or sieve. This just slightly whitens the meat. Do not overdip in boiling water or the delicate flavor will be lost forever! Drain.

Sprinkle 1 Tablespoon rice wine vinegar and MSG on chicken. Put aside. Sprinkle salt and 1 Tablespoon rice wine vinegar on cucumbers. Mix well. After 5 minutes squeeze out all moisture from cucumbers.

Combine and mix together seasoned chicken, cucumbers, *wasabi*, soy sauce, sugar and MSG. Sprinkle crushed toasted *nori* on top of this dish just before serving.

Lotus Nibbles *(Japanese)*

Top of stove   *Serves many*

When fresh lotus root (*renkon*) is available despite the expensive price here in America try this crisp, crunchy and a definitely different lacy looking vegetable. It looks like large pieces of water hyacinth roots and grows in segments. When these roots are cut you will be delightfully surprised at the pure white sections full of small holes.

Peel 1 or 2 lengths of *renkon* roots. Wash. Slice in paper thin slices. Wash again to remove some of the stickiness. Place slices in a saucepan. Cover with cold water. Parboil 2 minutes on high heat. *Renkon* will be crisp. Drain off liquid.

Put hot *renkon* in a small bowl. Pour rice wine vinegar to cover. Let stand for 30 minutes. Drain off this vinegar.

Mix the following dressing and marinate at least 1 hour before serving. Keeps in a bottle under refrigeration for days.

> **6 teaspoons rice wine vinegar**
> **3 teaspoons sugar**
> **1 teaspoon water**
> **dashes MSG (optional) and salt**

Since everyone's taste buds work differently you may wish to increase slightly the amount of sugar in this recipe. Sprinkle a bit more when you taste it prior to serving. Mix well to dissolve.

Optional method of using lotus root: This is one of the favorite ways and most unusual methods of preparation for Westerners. Slice the lotus root in thin chips and then deep-fry. Drain on paper towels and sprinkle a dash of salt. Crunchy, different and very popular for nibbling! Indescribable flavor! Don't overeat or your weight control plans will go flying away!

Tofu Teriyaki Bites *(Japanese)*

Top of stove and broiler   *Serves many*

This type of *tofu* is not available in all stores as yet. However in time more stores will begin to specialize so keep looking and asking. This brown colored *tofu* is not *age* which is deep-fried and very oily by comparison. I refer to *nama yaki dofu*.

Sauce:
   2 Tablespoons sherry wine
   1 teaspoon cornstarch
   2 Tablespoons soy sauce *(shoyu)*
   ½ teaspoon fresh ginger root, grated
   1 clove garlic, smashed
   1 ½ Tablespoons brown sugar, packed in spoon to measure
   ¼ teaspoon dry mustard powder
   dash MSG (optional)

Boil above ingredients for a few minutes until thickened. Cool. Use as marinade.

   1 raw fried soy bean cake *(nama yaki dofu)*
   green onions, chopped for garnish
   3 Tablespoons white sesame seeds, toasted and crushed for garnish

Marinate raw fried *tofu* for 1 hour. Turn over once. Place *tofu* on a pan and broil for 1 minute on each side. Baste with balance of sauce. Cut into ¾ inch pieces. Garnish with sesame seeds and onions. Serve hot with toothpicks.

Chicken Salad *(Chinese)*

Oven

This most unusual salad will banish boredom in your dull "same old" salad syndrome. It is more of an entrée than salad in the Western sense. But since lettuce is being used we most often term it in the salad type classification.

2 large chicken breasts with skin or 4–5 large thighs
Ingredients A:
    1 ½ Tablespoons soy sauce *(shoyu)*
    1 Tablespoon oil
    ½ teaspoon sugar
    1 Tablespoon sherry wine
    1 Tablespoon *hoisin* sauce (vegetable sauce)
    ½ clove garlic, minced
    1 Tablespoon fresh ginger root, grated
    1 teaspoon sesame oil
    1 teaspoon dry mustard powder
    ½ teaspoon salt
    dashes MSG (optional) and Chinese 5-spice powder

Soak chicken in ingredients A overnight. If chicken is icy cold direct from refrigerator allow to stand in room temperature for 45 minutes prior to baking. Preheat oven at 400°F. for 15 minutes. Put chicken in baking pan. Roast a total of 35 minutes turning occasionally until browned and meat portion is done. Do not overcook or it will be dry. Broil a minute or two if necessary to further brown skin and meat. Any left-over marinade can be brushed on chicken a minute before removing from oven.

Cool chicken. Pull pieces of chicken from bone. Cut meat and skin into matchstick size lengths. Remove extra fat from drippings in baking pan. Add a little hot water to loosen the crusted tasty portions stuck on pan. Add ½ teaspoon dry mustard into this juice. Add slivers of chicken, mix and scrape up all the good flavors.

Prepare the following ingredients in little mounds. Just before serving combine everything by tossing loosely in a large salad bowl. Do not allow to stand too long or the special delightful crunchiness will be destroyed. Garnish with Chinese parsley.

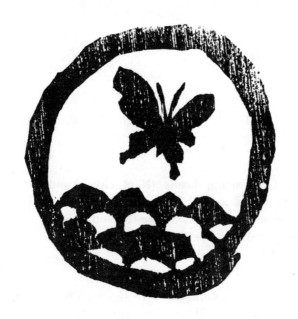

3 Tablespoons sweet pickles or pickled scallions *(rakkyo)*, **slivered thin**
3 stalks green onions, green and white portions, shredded
half a head of iceberg lettuce, shredded (about 2 cups)
2 Tablespoons Chinese parsley, coarsely minced
¼ cup salted peanuts, no skins, chopped
¼ cup toasted white sesame seeds
a few handfuls of deep-fried rice sticks *(mai-fun)*, **crumbled just before mixing into salad**
3 Tablespoons Chinese green sweet pickled cucumbers *(cha gwa)*, **slivered (optional)**

How to fry rice sticks: Loosen up rice sticks on a plate. Make up portions of small handfuls ready for frying. Heat oil to 350°F. as for deep frying. A Chinese wok is ideal for this since its high sides allow little spatter of oil. Drop a small handful at once into oil and almost instantly the rice sticks will puff up. Turn if necessary. Drain well on paper towels. Rice sticks will appear white, puffed and be very crisp if the heat temperature was correct. Have paper towels ready since the frying stage is a matter of seconds. A pair of tongs is fine for this operation of removing rice sticks in speedy fashion.

Goma Ae *(Japanese)*

Top of stove *Serves 4*

This recipe takes cold cooked vegetables out of "ordinary" to "gourmet" levels. See if you do not agree with me?

> ½ **pound fresh string beans (Kentucky Wonders are especially ideal if available), wash, cut ends and string**
> 1 ½ **Tablespoons sesame seeds, toasted and crushed**
> 1 **Tablespoon soy sauce** *(shoyu)*
> 2 **teaspoons sugar**
> **dash MSG (optional)**

Slice prepared string beans diagonally in 1 ½ inch pieces. Parboil without salt for about 5–8 minutes. Just enough to be tender but still crunchy. Drain.

Blend balance of ingredients together and mix with the cooked string beans. Serve at room temperature.

Variations: Other vegetables can be substituted such as spinach, carrots, lettuce leaves slightly parboiled, etc.

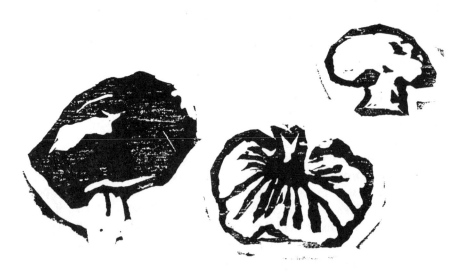

Special Turkey

Oven *Serves 4*

An entirely different method of using the flavored stock from preparing Chinese Pot Roast (page 15). I have found that this method is one way to use the wonderful flavors of the juices blended with so many goodies. Turkey meat generally when roasted is so dry—this will be flavorsome and most succulent. And with turkey so easily available and most reasonably priced—you should try it soon.

> **2 hindquarters of turkey (about 4 pounds), 2 legs and 2 thighs**
> **about 1 cup of the flavored stock from cooking Chinese Pot Roast**
> **1 Tablespoon honey**
> **½ teaspoon Chinese 5-spice powder**
> **several sprigs of Chinese parsley**
> **dashes of salt, garlic salt and MSG(optional)**

Place turkey in a roasting pan with the skin side up. Sprinkle with salt, garlic salt and MSG(optional). Roast in preheated oven 350°F. for about 15 minutes to brown skin slightly. Pour in the remainder of ingredients over the turkey. Periodically baste turkey with same. As it roasts you will find that the honey makes for very good browning of the surfaces.

The resulting meat will be especially moist if you turn over the meat at least once during the roasting process and make a few slits in the flesh. Baste some more. About 1 hour or 1¼ hours will complete the baking time required. This is a simple method of preparation and can be either eaten cold or hot. You could even make it the day before. It is most delightful sliced cold also. A garnish of Chinese parsley is most appropriate for this dish.

Kim Pira *(Japanese)*

Top of stove   *Serves many*

This spicy burdock (*gobo*) adds zip to your meal and can be made ahead. Serve at room temperature. Excellent as an appetizer to be nibbled and nibbled.

>**2 cups burdock roots, peeled, washed, shredded or shaved
>   very thin. About ½ dozen small roots will be enough**
>**1 small carrot, shredded thin**
>**1 Tablespoon oil**
>**2 Tablespoons soy sauce *(shoyu)***
>**2 Tablespoons sugar**
>**dash MSG (optional)**
>**¼ teaspoon dried crushed chili pepper or substitute
>   several dashes cayenne pepper**

Soak burdock and carrots in slightly salted water to prevent oxidation. When ready to cook, drain well. Heat skillet on moderate heat. Add oil. Fry vegetables for about 5–7 minutes. Stir constantly. Add balance of ingredients. Complete frying process another 5 minutes until all flavorings are well absorbed.

This is a crunchy tid-bit and uses burdock, a root vegetable, which in the United States has been considered a nuisance weed. It is being cultivated and sold more commonly in specialized markets. Burdock is like a carrot and can be used in similar fashion. However, after peeling soak in salted water to prevent darkening. It never gets mushy even if slightly overcooked and has firmness of texture.

Entrées

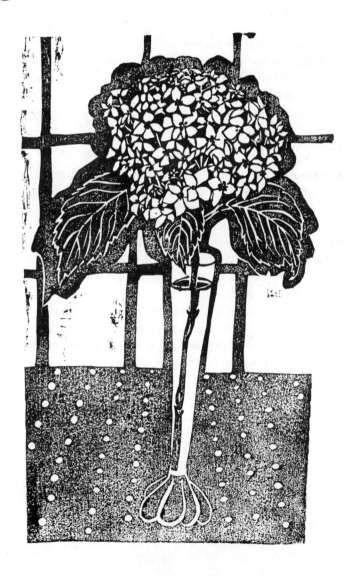

Fragrant Shrimp *(Japanese)*

Broiler or *hibachi*   *Serves 4*

Juicy morsels of shellfish. Very delicate in flavor with a delicious difference. Again, quick and easy!

> **24 large shrimp**
> **Ingredients A:**
>   **2 egg yolks, slightly beaten**
>   **2 Tablespoons *mirin* (Japanese sweet rice wine) or**
>   **sherry (if using sherry add 1 teaspoon sugar to make**
>   **it more like *mirin*)**
>   **1 teaspoon lemon juice**
>   **½ teaspoon salt**
>   **dashes MSG (optional)**

Wash shrimp removing the legs. Leave the shells intact. If desired the
back vein can be removed by inserting a sharp knife blade slightly therein through shell and scraping vein out onto a paper towel.

Make a slit on the underside of shrimp where legs were removed.
Open flat and with the blade of your cleaver flatten the flesh lightly.
Thread the shrimp onto skewers. Soaking wooden skewers prior to use
in water for 15 minutes so that they will be water-logged will prevent
burning over the hot coals.

Mix ingredients A until well blended. Brush this mixture on the meat
portion of the shrimp. Broil over charcoal with the shell portion down,
turning over and periodically basting with the remaining sauce, if any.
Broil only a total of 3 minutes or less.

Cabbage Rolls *(Japanese)*

Top of stove   *Serves 4*

This is one of the basic manners of preparing dishes in Japan. Cooking in broth. Traditionally a seaweed and fish base stock called *dashi* is used. However, I suggest you start with chicken broth and after a more experienced palate develops try *dashi*. This is definitely a fat-free method of cooking and can be achieved with simple cooking facilities.

> **8 leaves removed from a large head of Chinese cabbage (*nappa*)**
> **Ingredients A:**
> **2 cups minced chicken meat or substitute ground lean pork**
> **½ cup bread crumbs or 3 slices white bread, crumbled**
> **1 egg**
> **1 teaspoon salt**
> **dashes pepper**
> **dash MSG (optional)**

Blanch cabbage leaves in plenty of boiling water for 2 minutes–just long enough to wilt them. Mix ingredients A until well blended. Make 8 balls with the mixture and place them on the cabbage leaves. Roll up cabbage like packets. Fold over the ends so that the meat balls will not come out during the cooking process.

Put following ingredients into a shallow pan with cover. Arrange packets in bottom of pan and simmer for 15 minutes.

> **1 cup chicken broth**
> **⅓ cup sherry wine**
> **3 Tablespoons light soy sauce *(shoyu)***
> **3 Tablespoons sugar**

Remove cabbage packets carefully onto a platter. Thicken the remaining juices with 1½ Tablespoons cornstarch dissolved in 2 Tablespoons water. Pour this gravy over cabbage rolls.

Shabu-Shabu *(Japanese Fondue)*

Table top cooking   *Serves 4*

This meal can be cooked at the table with ease. Have each diner place his desired ingredients into the bubbling broth to cook to his desired doneness one or two pieces at a time. This is excellent for cold winter nights since the bubbling soup in the pan gives off heat and warms your insides at the same time. And what a marvelous way to get to know each other better. You may be "stuck" with your dinner partners for several hours with this manner of cookery! Superb food enjoyed in an atmosphere that lingers on long after a meal is a wonderful memory!

> **8 cups chicken broth flavored with dashes MSG, salt, sherry and 2 Tablespoons lemon juice**
> **2 cups boneless chicken meat, sliced thin strips**
> **2 cups tender lean beef, sliced thin and rolled like cigarettes**
> **1 large block of soy bean cake *(tofu)*, cut 1 inch square cubes**
> **1 medium-sized Chinese cabbage *(nappa)*, cut 2 inch square pieces**
> **1 bunch green onions, sliced diagonally 2 inch pieces**
> **1 large carrot, cut decoratively into thin flower shapes, if possible**
> **1 bunch edible chrysanthemum *(shungiku)*, cut 2 inch pieces (optional)**
> **1 can *shirataki* (yam noodles) or substitute mung bean threads *(sai fun)*, soaked in hot water for 20 minutes and cut in 2 inch lengths**
> **6 fresh mushrooms, sliced ¼ inch thickness**

Prepare all ingredients substituting, if necessary, with what you have on hand. And, again, seasonal availability will make a difference in what you can purchase at the market. Place everything artistically on platter near the electric skillet or fire pot that you have placed in the middle of the table filled with broth mixture. Let broth come to bubbling.

Each diner puts in what he would like to taste first. Generally, meat is done first and then the vegetables follow. Dip into one of the follow-

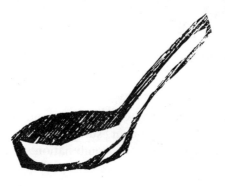

ing sauces as you complete each cooking process which takes only about 1 minute per bite! Place sauces in little dishes by each diner's plate.

For a change have several different dips. You will get exciting flavor variations. The following are interesting tastes but invent some of your own as time goes on:

Dipping Sauce #1
A simple dip can be made from equal parts soy sauce
(shoyu) and lemon juice plus puréed daikon radish.
An addition of Japanese green horseradish or fresh
ginger makes it even better

Dipping Sauce #2
2 Tablespoons toasted white sesame seeds, ground
4 Tablespoons soup stock
½ teaspoon dry mustard powder
2 Tablespoons white soy bean paste (shiro miso)
1 Tablespoon rice wine vinegar
½ teaspoon sugar
dashes MSG (optional)
dash salt

Blend altogether and dip morsels of hot ingredients from the *shabu-shabu*. Serve steamed rice in bowls. The remaining soup broth after all the cooking is completed is such a delicious ambrosia. Be sure to add some of the dipping sauce for added zest. Noodles could be cooked in the broth at the last. This will be a hearty and yet very light meal–surprisingly the ingredients will serve many persons prepared this way. I always precut too many vegetables so take a lesson from me–do not overly cut!

Kushiyaki *(Japanese)*

Broiler or *hibachi*   *Serves 4*

This skewered meat is a favorite with everyone and always a great "hit"
mainly because the tantalizing flavors suit practically all palates. I have
yet to hear of someone disliking this combination. So it is a safe bet for
you to serve anytime.

> **1½ pounds pork, cut 1 inch squares**
> **1 or 2 large green peppers, cut into 1 inch squares**
> **2 bunches green onions, cut into 2 inch lengths or substi-
> tute 8—10 tiny white boiling onions, left whole or cut in
> half**
> **2 medium size zucchini squash, unpeeled, cut into ¾ inch
> wide slices**

Spear meat and vegetables alternately on individual skewers. Marinate
in the following sauce for about ¾ hour at room temperature turning
a few times so flavors will penetrate.

> **Marinade:**
> **5 Tablespoons soy sauce *(shoyu)***
> **2 Tablespoons sugar**
> **2 teaspoons fresh ginger root, grated**
> **4 Tablespoons sherry wine**
> **dashes MSG (optional)**

Drain and use sauce for basting during broiling period. *Kushiyaki* is
best and tastiest when broiled over hot charcoals although your stove
broiler gives quite satisfactory results.

Note: If using wooden skewers soak them in water for a brief time
before use so they will not burn with the heat while broiling.

Ginger Pork *(Japanese)*

Top of stove   *Serves 4*

Delicious, attractive and quick to prepare. Pork is quite lean these days and not as fat as in years past. And a most nutritious food.

1 pound pork butt, sliced ⅛ × 2 × 3 inches
1 teaspoon oil
Ingredients A:
    2 Tablespoons soy sauce *(shoyu)*
    1 Tablespoon sugar
    2 Tablespoons fresh ginger root, grated
    1 Tablespoon sherry wine
    ½ small onion, chopped
    dash MSG (optional)

Marinate meat in ingredients A for 1 hour. Turn over once. Heat skillet or wok on high heat. Add oil. Slosh around. Sear pork slices. Brown on both sides about 7 minutes total time. Depends on meat thickness. Add green onions just before removing from pan. Cook about 1 minute after they have been added. Be sure pork is fully cooked with no pink color inside. Serve with rice and a vegetable dish for an easy balanced meal.

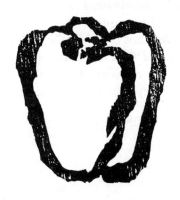

Barbecued Chicken *(Chinese)*

Broiler or *hibachi* *Serves 4*

Another chicken recipe but definitely worth trying since flavor is magnificent.

> **1 chicken fryer, about 3 pounds**
> **salt**
> **Marinade:**
> **¼ teaspoon Chinese 5-spice powder**
> **½ teaspoon fresh ginger root, grated**
> **1 clove garlic, minced**
> **2 teaspoons sugar**
> **2 teaspoons brown bean sauce (soy bean condiment)**
> **2 teaspoons red bean curd *(nam yoi)***
> **4 teaspoons *hoisin* sauce**
> **1 Tablespoon sherry wine**
> **2 Tablespoons soy sauce *(shoyu)***
> **⅓ cup oil**

Cut chicken into serving pieces such as wings, thighs, etc. Sprinkle with salt lightly. Blend marinade ingredients. Pour this sauce over chicken and marinate overnight or all day. If weather is not too hot keep at room temperature during marinating period. Occasionally spoon sauce on chicken and turn chicken around.

Barbecue chicken over hot coals for 20 or 30 minutes turning and basting frequently so that chicken is not dried out. This can be broiled in oven if hot coals are not convenient. Again I emphasize care in broiling. Do not overcook. Juicy morsels are so much tastier than dried out pieces. Cook with love!

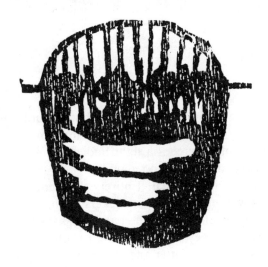

Yakitori (Japanese)

Broiler or *hibachi*   *Serves 4*

Actually a *teriyaki* type chicken. This will satisfy your guests with its special tantalizing flavor. Especially when they catch a whiff of the cooking aroma.

> **2 whole chicken breasts (about 1¾ pounds), cut meat into**
>   **1 inch chunks**
> **½ cup sherry or Japanese rice wine *(sake)***
> **½ cup soy sauce *(shoyu)***
> **2 Tablespoons sugar**
> **2 Tablespoons fresh ginger root, grated**
> **dash MSG (optional)**

Thread chicken on wooden skewers. Combine balance of ingredients in a small sauce pan and bring to boil. Simmer for about 15 minutes until sauce has been reduced in volume.

Preheat broiler or prepare your charcoal *hibachi*. Dip the chicken in sauce and broil for 2 or 3 minutes. Turn and brush marinade often while the chicken is broiling. A total of 5 or 6 minutes should be sufficient time to complete the broiling of the chicken. Brush with sauce just before serving on platter. Garnish with parsley.

45

Gyoza *(Japanese)*

Top of stove *Serves 4*

A stuffed dumpling originally Chinese but beautifully borrowed by the Japanese. This version uses relatively little meat in proportion to vegetables and truly stretches a tight budget. Low calorie and highly nutritious—if you do not eat too many!

This is a savory filled treat. Entirely different from dumplings as Westerners know them. Called pot stickers by the Chinese because they appear as if they would stick to the pan. And sometimes they do! However with a spatula they are easily lifted up to serve. The individual morsels are placed on a platter and served with a dipping sauce of your choice. These are a tasty and filling "one bite" and don't be surprised at the speed with which they are consumed. Make plenty.

> **Ingredients A:**
> **¾ pound Chinese cabbage or substitute spinach or *bok choy***
> **1 cup ground pork meat**
> **1 stalk green onion, chopped**
> **½ teaspoon fresh ginger root, grated**
> **1 clove garlic, minced**
> **¾ teaspoon salt**
> **1 Tablespoon soy sauce *(shoyu)***
> **1 Tablespoon cornstarch**
> **1 Tablespoon sherry wine**
> **1 Tablespoon oil**
> **2 teaspoons sesame oil**
> **dash MSG (optional)**
> **1 pound package of *gyoza* or round skins (about 70—80 sheets). Wrap well and freeze any skins which you do not use since you will need less than half for this recipe**

Or if you cannot secure the prepared skins make your own as follows:

> **3 cups flour**
> **dashes salt**
> **1 cup hot water**

Make filling by blanching cabbage. Dip into boiling water a few seconds. Drain. Chop fine and remove excess water. Add ingredients A altogether. Mix well to blend flavorings. Put this filling aside while you prepare the skin. Add hot water to flour and salt mixture. Mix well. Knead dough until smooth and elastic on a well-floured board. Cover with a damp cloth (not dripping!) and let dough rest for 30 minutes.

Roll on a floured board 2 inch diameter long rolls of dough. Slice off ¾ inch slices. Flatten each piece with the palm of the hand. Make skins about 4 × ⅛ inch thick. Use rolling pin with right hand while you turn skin with left hand.

Place about 2 teaspoons filling on center of dough round. Dab water on edges. Bring opposite sides of skin together like a half moon. Flute and pinch one side onto the other making sure that it seals well. If you cannot do this very well simply press the two sides like a miniature tart.

Use hot oiled skillet. Arrange dumplings in rows to fry until golden brown about 4 minutes. Add hot water or some chiken broth about ⅓ of the height of dumplings. Cover and steam-fry over medium heat until liquid evaporates. Use spatula to remove. Serve browned side up on platter. Dip in soy sauce, mustard and vinegar as you eat for additional flavor.

These can be just boiled in water, drained and served with the sauce. To give zip try using Szechwan chili paste—you will be surprised at the fantastic hot flavor—hotter than all the chili in Texas! And still with a different taste entirely. Try some soon.

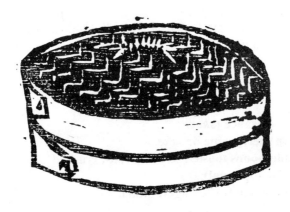

Karibayaki *(Japanese)*

Table top cooking   *Serves 4*

This recipe has everyone participating in the preparation of the foods. That alone will make persons feel so very important. To make an Asian-style meal without much work! As the hostess you will have to just precut the meat and vegetables. You can enjoy your own party.

One can use an electric grill, skillet or Genghis Khan domed grill. This last mentioned utensil is available in many gourmet shops these days. It has proven to me to be most adapable for the American's casual way of life. I place my domed utensil on top of the *hibachi* coals. There are grooves with a few holes here and there. The grooves direct the juices from cooking toward the rim of the pan. There I often place the smaller vegetables to absorb the delightful juices as they drip downward. It will be the center of attraction if you can find one. And definitely place your dinner on a pedestal since it will be so spectacular.

> ½ **pound beef (*sukiyaki* meat, sirloin, tenderloin or market steak), sliced thin in 3 inch square pieces**
> ½ **pound chicken breast or thigh, sliced thin**
> **1 pound medium-sized mushrooms, sliced ¼ inch thick**
> **2 bunches green onions, cut into 2 inch lengths (diagonally cut for attractiveness)**
> **2 large sweet dry onions, sliced in ¼ inch slices (halve if too large)**

Arrange the above ingredients individually and in artistic manner on plates for each diner. Place about ½ cup of the following sauce in a little dish at each place serving. Raw egg could be in another bowl if your diners are the adventurous types.

> **Sauce:**
> **1 cup soy sauce *(shoyu)***
> ¾ **cup sherry wine or *sake***
> **2 Tablespoons toasted sesame seeds, crushed**
> **dash msg (optional)**
> **1 Tablespoon fresh ginger, grated**

Put a piece of suet in whatever utensil you are going to use or pat some with a brush on cooking surface. When pan is hot each person should dip the piece of meat and vegetable he desires into sauce and cook them to his own taste. The food will be very hot to eat directly from pan but it is both cooled and improved in flavor by dipping into the raw, slightly beaten egg just before eating. The heat will partially cook the rawness out of egg. It is far more tasty than it might sound. Here is another good dipping sauce in place of the raw egg:

1 cup Japanese *daikon* radish, puréed
1½ Tablespoons soy sauce *(shoyu)*
1 or 2 Tablespoons stock or *dashi*
a pinch of Japanese red pepper *(togarashi)*
dash MSG (optional)

Bowls of hot steaming rice go well with this *karibayaki*. A few salted Japanese pickles or sliced kosher dills are good additions to this meal.

Delicate Broiled Fish *(Japanese)*

Broiler or *hibachi*   *Serves 4*

This manner of plain simple broiling is much appreciated in Japan. The true fish flavor is clear and unadulterated. If fish is small and left whole, slash 3 diagonal cuts on the scaled skin of fish on both sides. Lightly sprinkle with salt. Allow to stand 30 minutes for penetration of salt.

If fillets are used there is no need to slash surfaces. Broil about 4 minutes under preheated broiler. Turn over and broil for 5 minutes on other side. Serve with lemon wedges. Soy sauce *(shoyu)* plus a small mound of puréed *daikon* radish goes well with this.

One of the choicest fish made this way is sardine. However, on our Pacific coast shores we no longer can get this elegant tasting fish. The schools of fish that inhabited Monterey Bay have disappeared but hopefully some year in the future they will return to their original habitat.

This is definitely a non-fattening method of fish cookery and a mode of cooking that you should certainly try.

Batayaki *(Japanese)*

Table top cooking   *Serves 4*

Favorite ingredients team up to make this dish extra easy to prepare since the cook only gets the ingredients cut ahead of time. The diners can make their own or if the hostess wishes she can do the honors in front of the guests. Many steak houses are becoming popular using this same method of cooking. Their main attraction is the skillful manner and acting on the part of the chef. This could come with some practice on your part. So get that bit of "ham" out working in you. And after it is all over you can deservedly bow to your fascinated audience.

> **1 pound prime rib boneless roast, Spencer steaks or fillet**
> **beef, sliced about ¼ inch thick**
> **2 onions, sliced ½ inch thick**
> **1 pound fresh mushrooms, sliced ⅜ inch thick**
> **1 bunch fresh spinach or Chinese cabbage (nappa)**
> **½ pound fresh bean sprouts, washed and drained**
> **2 bunches green onions, cut into 1½ inch lengths**
> **½ cube (⅛ pound) butter**

Heat electric skillet or grill to high. Add pat of butter and a portion of meat and vegetables. Salt slightly while frying. Sauté quickly and serve while piping hot. Keep crisp. Eat by dipping in sauce made with the following ingredients:

> **½ cup soy sauce *(shoyu)***
> **½ cup lemon juice or rice wine vinegar**
> **2 Tablespoons sugar**
> **½ teaspoon MSG (optional)**

Or, you may wish to try another zippy flavored sauce:

> **2 teaspoons dry mustard**
> **6 Tablespoons soy sauce *(shoyu)***

Dissolve mustard in small amount of water. Mix with soy. Serve in dipping dishes.

Condiments to add flourish to the sauce can be chosen from the following: green onions (finely chopped), grated fresh ginger root,

50

crushed toasted sesame seeds, Japanese *daikon* radish (puréed) or laver seaweed (*nori*), toasted and crumbled.

Other meats and vegetables can be substituted very easily since the various food ingredients are not interdependent upon each other for additional flavor. You savor each individual piece by itself. Suggestions: oysters, shrimp, scallops, chicken meat, pork, lamb, etc. Chinese snow peas (edible pod peas), green peppers, string beans (Kentucky Wonders ideal), small eggplants, summer squash, etc.

Asparagus with Velvet Sauce (Japanese)

Top of stove   *Serves 4*

In the bright clear days of spring when the first asparagus comes to market try this recipe. It will be such a different experience and you will find the flavors mingle subtly.

> **1 pound asparagus, trimmed and parboiled briefly—do not overcook (probably about 5 minutes is more than enough)**
> **2 Tablespoons sugar**
> **2 Tablespoons *shiro miso* (white soy bean paste)**
> **5 Tablespoons rice wine vinegar**
> **¼ teaspoon MSG (optional)**

Blend sugar and *miso* well. Add vinegar and MSG and stir. This will have an appearance of a heavy salad dressing. (It could serve as an addition to your salad repertoire.)

Attractively arrange asparagus on individual salad plates. Pour sauce in a neat line across the spears. Do it carefully so the final appearance will look enticing. A garnish of a yellow flower or sieved hard boiled egg yolk would be good.

Fresh string beans, broccolli, cauliflower, green onions, etc. are all good substitute vegetables. Vegetables could be slightly parboiled until tender and crisp. Seafoods such as clams, crab and shrimp lend themselves well with this sauce. Try the sauce alone on shredded iceberg lettuce. This is fairly low in calories.

51

Chinese Omelet

Top of stove *Serves many*

Prepare the filling first and set aside while you make the omelet. This will be something like egg *foo young* but perhaps simpler to make.

> **1 cup raw shrimp, shelled, deveined and cut into small pieces or substitute 1 can shrimp or crab, drained**
> **½ cup Oriental dried mushrooms *(shiitake)*, soaked in warm water, squeezed and sliced thin**
> **½ pound fresh mung bean sprouts, washed and well drained**
> **1 small onion, halved and cut in thin slices**
> **1 rib of celery, slashed into thin layers and then sliced diagonally to make paper-thin slivers**
> **½ teaspoon fresh ginger root, grated**
> **¾ teaspoon salt (adjust if you use canned shellfish since usually it is quite salty already)**
> **dash MSG (optional)**
> **1 Tablespoon soy sauce *(shoyu)***
> **dash sugar**
> **8 eggs, slightly beaten**
> **3 Tablespoons oil for frying**

Heat skillet or wok on high heat. Add 1 Tablespoon oil. Slosh around. Add shrimp and all ingredients except eggs and oil. Fry about 3 minutes to heat through. Vegetables should be slightly crisp tender. Put aside in warm oven while you make the omelets.

Clean skillet. Add some of the oil reserved for frying. Slosh around. Pour about a third of the egg mixture into skillet. Make an omelet without allowing it to get too browned. Use medium heat. Cook 1 or 2 minutes, running spatula around edge of egg mixture to let uncooked portion run underneath. Place a third of the cooked shrimp and vegetable mixture across center of omelet. Fold right side of omelet over filling then overlap with left side of omelet, sliding onto a warmed platter. Keep in warm oven while you prepare the next omelet. Repeat process.

Make sauce before you begin the frying so that it can be ready immediately upon completion of the omelet preparation.

Sauce ingredients:
  1½ teaspoons soy sauce
  2 teaspoons cornstarch
  ½ teaspoon sugar
  dash MSG (optional)
  salt if desired
  ½ cup juice from shrimp drained from can plus water
    or broth only

Mix all sauce ingredients and cook until thickened. Pour over the filled omelets and garnish with chopped green onions.

Eggplant with Meat Sauce (Japanese)

Top of stove   *Serves 4*

A marvelous fresh new use for eggplant—the "meat" substitute vegetable. Even eggplant "haters" will love it.

  1 large eggplant or 8 medium Japanese type eggplants
  1 Tablespoon oil
  1 cup very lean beef, ground (such a round or sirloin)
  3 Tablespoons white soy bean paste *(shiro miso)*
  1 teaspoon fresh ginger root, grated
  1 Tablespoon sugar
  1 Tablespoon sherry wine
  2 Tablespoons stock or water
  . dash MSG (optional)
  dash *shichimi* pepper (optional)

Slice large eggplant without peeling into ¼ inch rounds. Leave Japanese type eggplant partially cut towards calyx and making criss cross slashes on sides.

  Heat skillet over medium heat. Add oil. Fry until tender about 3 or 4 minutes. Remove to warm platter. If skillet is not oily enough, add a few drops oil. Then fry meat. Add balance of ingredients blending well. Cook about 3 minutes. Pour over prepared eggplant. Garnish with a few chopped green onions.

53

Beef Glazed *(Japanese)*

Top of stove *Serves 4*

This goes together fast and is a fine entrée that teams nicely with perhaps a vegetable and salad to round out a meal. And as mentioned before you do not have to make it an Asian menu. It is a good combination with any meal.

2 pounds beef, rib eye steaks or fillet, sliced ¼ inch thick
piece of suet
Ingredients A:
    4 Tablespoons sherry wine
    3 Tablespoons soy sauce *(shoyu)*
    1 Tablespoon sugar
    dash MSG (optional)
    1 teaspoon fresh ginger root, grated

Heat skillet on high heat. Add suet. Allow fat to be rendered a few minutes. Remove suet. Put steak pieces into hot skillet. Sear to brown meat quickly on both sides.

Add ingredients A over meat. Heat on high heat only about ½ minute more for sauce to penetrate slightly. Place a small mound of grated ginger or Japanese horseradish (*wasabi*) by the meat. Serve immediately.

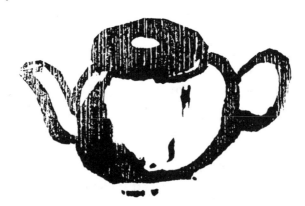

Dry Curried Rice *(Japanese)*

Top of stove *Serves 4*

An entirely novel way for curry to appear in a rice dish. A ½ cup of rice is only 100 calories so along with the other "goodies" in this dish adding a few more calories you can slowly savor every kernel. A terrific way to use left-over rice and it will not taste like left-overs. In fact you might wish to make some rice on purpose for this dish. Be sure that it is refrigerated and cold before starting this recipe.

> ¼ **pound lean ground beef**
> **2 onions, chopped fine**
> ½ **medium size carrot, grated fine**
> **1 Tablespoon oil for frying**
> **Ingredients A:**
>   **1 Tablespoon light soy sauce** *(shoyu)*
>   **1 teaspoon sugar**
>   **1 teaspoon salt**
>   **1½ teaspoons curry powder or more**
>   **dashes pepper and MSG (optional)**
>   **6 cups cold cooked rice**

Heat skillet on high heat. Add oil. Slosh around. Add ground beef. Stir. Add onions and carrots. Fry about 3 minutes stirring all the while so that there will be no sticking. While everything is cooking add ingredients A. Mix altogether thoroughly so ingredients will be well harmonized. Fry until everything is completely heated through. Taste and adjust seasonings if desired. It can be made ahead and reheated.

Spanish Mackerel with Ginger *(Japanese)*

Top of stove   *Serves 4*

Spanish mackerel is a tasty fish available fresh in most world markets. The main identification mark of this fish is the peculiar scale pattern. A single line of scales goes along the side of the fish body—one on each side. This method of cooking fish could be adapted to other types of fish especially the fattier types such as salmon, sea bass, etc.

Fish has a higher water content than meat therefore the flavor of fish is more delicate. As it is well known fish protein is nutritionally interchangeable with that of meat. The percentage of protein, ounce for ounce, is the same.

> **4 small size Spanish mackerel *(aji)* or similar fatty fish with skin intact, scaled. If fish is large, cut up into appropriate individual serving pieces. Total weight of fish should be about 2 pounds**
> **dashes salt**
> **⅓ cup water or broth**
> **4 Tablespoons *mirin* (sweet rice wine) or sherry wine**
> **4 Tablespoons soy sauce *(shoyu)*, or less**
> **2 Tablespoons sugar**
> **dash MSG (optional)**
> **2 large leeks, cut 1½ inch lengths, diagonally**
> **1½ Tablespoons fresh ginger root, grated**
> **1 stalk green onions, chopped**

Sprinkle fish with salt. Let stand for 1 hour. Place water, *mirin* and fish in shallow pan. Simmer 10 minutes without stirring. Add soy sauce, sugar, MSG and leeks. Continue simmering about 5 more minutes. Baste with juices occasionally. Remove and arrange attractively on individual plates for serving. Garnish with grated ginger and chopped green onions. If desired a small piece of ginger root could be used for the simmering period for added flavor.

Scrambled Eggs with Beans *(Japanese)*

Top of stove   *Serves 4*

This recipe will be a revelation to you that here again is still another way to make eggs taste entirely different from breakfast eggs. And with such a good source of inexpensive protein you will enjoy this recipe much.

> ¼ **pound raw shrimp, shelled, deveined, washed and chopped fine**
> ½ **pound fresh string beans, washed, strings removed, cut ¾ inch diagonally**
> **1 Tablespoon oil for frying**
> **6 eggs, slightly beaten**
> **2 teaspoons soy sauce *(shoyu)***
> ½ **teaspoon salt**
> **1½ teaspoons sugar**
> **dash MSG (optional)**

Heat skillet on medium heat. Add oil. Fry shrimp and beans for 5 minutes until crunchy tender. If necessary add a tablespoon or two of water to prevent scorching. Keep mixing all the time.

Mix eggs with soy, salt, sugar and MSG. Pour this egg mixture over beans and shrimp. Scramble lightly after partially set. Do not use high heat since this would toughen the egg. The resultant egg combination should be soft and coddled. Not dry and flaky.

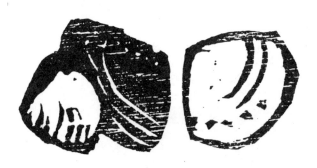

Different Sweet and Sour Ribs *(Chinese)*

Top of stove   *Serves 4*

A simplified method of preparing this dish results in no oil used in the recipe. (Generally sweet and sour pork is deep-fried in quantities of oil, drained and combined with sauce). This allows you to enjoy the subtleness of the sweet and tart flavors. If eaten in moderation you will be on safe territory!

> **1½ pounds pork spareribs, cut into small 1 inch square pieces. Choose small, lean pork ribs since they are the most tender**
> **1 cup boiling water**
> **1 clove garlic, peel removed**
> **1 inch square piece of fresh ginger root**
> **1 teaspoon salt**
> **3 Tablespoons cider vinegar**
> **dash MSG (optional)**

Simmer the above ingredients covered for 30 minutes. Test to see if meat is tender otherwise continue to cook a little longer. Remove ribs with a skimmer to another dish. Discard garlic and ginger pieces. Skim off excess fat from the pork-vinegar water that ribs were cooked in. Reserve this liquid for use in sauce preparation.

> **½ large bulb onion, cut into chunks with 1 inch sides, separate layers**
> **1 rib celery, cut in chunks as above**
> **1 green pepper, cut in chunks as above**
> **1 cup pineapple chunks, drained**

Cook onion, celery, green pepper and pineapple in ½ cup pork-vinegar stock for 2 minutes.

Ingredients A:
⅓ cup pineapple juice
3 Tablespoons cider vinegar
7 Tablespoons brown sugar, packed down
2 Tablespoons catsup
1½ Tablespoons cornstarch
a few drops of red food coloring if reddish shade desired
   (optional)
a few drops tabasco sauce (optional)
dash MSG (optional)

Mix ingredients A in a small bowl. Add to pan with cooked vegetables and pork-vinegar stock. Blend well. Keep stirring over medium heat until thickened. Taste to see if you might wish to add a wee bit more vinegar or sugar. Add cooked ribs at this point and bring sauce up to boiling point to heat ribs completely.

Keep stirring so there will not be any scorching.

Optional: Serve over a bed of iceberg lettuce sliced thin like coleslaw. And without knowing it "almost" you have your salad built right in with your meal. Garnish with a few maraschino cherries, if available, for a contrast of color.

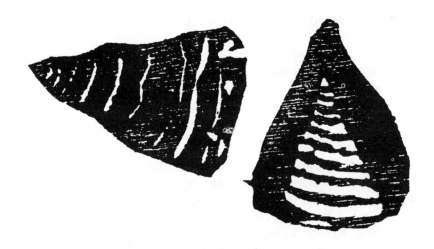

Soy Bean Sprouts with Pork *(Chinese)*

Top of stove *Serves 4*

Soy bean sprouts have large beans at one end of the sprout as compared to mung bean sprouts which have "wee" size beans attached. Naturally this is one of the most nutritious ways to consume soy beans. And when the beans are sprouted in this manner they present an increased amount of vitamin, mineral and protein as compared to eating the soy beans alone. You will begin to find more and more soy bean sprouts in the supermarkets since Westerners are "discovering" what has been known to Asians for centuries......the miraculous soy bean!

1 pound lean pork, cut in thin slices
2 Tablespoons oil for frying
1½ teaspoons fresh ginger root, grated
1 clove garlic, minced fine
1 pound soy bean sprouts (large beans attached to sprouts), washed and drained
1 small onion, halved, sliced in thin strips
½ cup edible pod peas (Chinese snow peas)
Ingredients A:
    1 teaspoon sugar
    1 teaspoon soy sauce *(shoyu)*
    1 teaspoon salt
    ¼ teaspoon pepper
    2 teaspoons cornstarch dissolved in ¼ cup water or chicken broth
    1 Tablespoon sherry wine
    1 teaspoon sesame oil
    dash MSG (optional)

Measure all ingredients A together before starting to cook.

Heat skillet or wok on high heat. Add 1 Tablespoon oil. Slosh around. Add soy bean sprouts, onion and celery. Salt slightly. Toss-fry about 2 minutes. Remove to platter.

Clean pan. Reheat on high heat. Add remaining 1 Tablespoon oil. Slosh around. Add ginger, garlic and pork making sure ginger and garlic hit the hot oil first. Toss-fry until meat is whitish. Add precooked vegetables, peas and ingredients A to the meat. Toss-fry for about 2 minutes until the cornstarch mixture has become translucent and and thickened. Taste adjusting salt if more is desired.

Stuffed Cucumbers *(Chinese)*

Top of stove–steamer   *Serves 4*

Asians use cucumbers as a cooked vegetable prepared in soups and entrées as well as raw in salad type dishes. It has the texture of slight crunchiness and yet soft to a degree. Cucumbers especially when they become overgrown and full of seeds can be cooked very nicely with seeds removed.

> **4 medium size cucumbers or zucchini squash (6—7-inches long), do not peel**
> **Ingredients A:**
> > **¾ pound lean pork, ground**
> > **1 small can (about ½ cup) water chestnuts, chopped fine**
> > **1 bunch green onions, minced fine**
> > **1 clove garlic, minced**
> > **1 teaspoon fresh ginger root, grated**
> > **2 teaspoons soy sauce *(shoyu)***
> > **1 teaspoon sugar**
> > **1 teaspoon cornstarch**
> > **¾ teaspoon salt**
> > **dash MSG (optional)**

Cut cucumbers lengthwise in half. Remove seeds. This makes a hollow-boat shaped vegetable. Combine ingredients A. Mound the mixture into cucumber cavity. Steam in a shallow baking pan such as a pie dish for 30 minutes. Be sure you have plenty of free flowing steam circulating around the dish. Serve the juices with the stuffed vegetables.

Try assorted vegetables such as Chinese cabbage (*nappa*) leaves blanched 2 minutes and cooled. Make a packet by placing a meat ball inside each leaf. Then leaf is rolled and tucked under.

Beef in Foil *(Chinese)*

Oven   *Serves 4*

Heavenly food suited for the Gods especially when served piping hot
from the oven. Usually this is prepared by deep fat frying but this
method is simpler and far less fattening! Easy too.

> **1 pound beef such as sirloin, fillet or other tender cuts,
>   sliced thin across grain ⅛ inch thickness**
> **1 teaspoon sugar**
> **1 Tablespoon soy sauce *(shoyu)***
> **1½ Tablespoons *hoisin* sauce**
> **1 Tablespoon sherry wine**
> **1 Tablespoon cornstarch**
> **3 stalks green onions, cut ¾ inch lengths**
> **2 Tablespoons fresh Chinese parsley (coriander), chopped**

Mix all ingredients. Divide into 4 portions. Carefully spread out
ingredients over the center of 4 pieces of foil (12 inches square). Wrap
either regular drug store wrap by making a double seal at the seam or
fold envelope style.

Bring D to B and C over to A. A over to C and finally seal by bring-
ing B over to D and tuck inside flap. Place with seams at top on a
baking sheet so your juices will not escape. Bake in a preheated 450°F.
oven for 6—7 minutes. Be sure to have steaming hot bowls of rice with
this.

Envelope Style Wrap

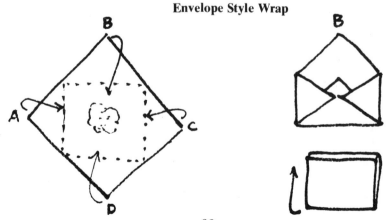

62

Drug Store Style Wrap

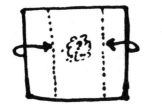 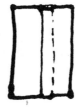

"Hot" Bean Cakes *(Chinese)*

Top of stove   *Serves 4*

Epicurean seasoned dash of "fire" makes this a most unusual dish. A calorie counter's special.

1 Tablespoon oil for frying
¼ pound ground lean pork
2 stalks green onions, chopped
½ teaspoon fresh ginger root, grated
1 clove garlic, smashed, minced fine
½ teaspoon red chili pepper flakes (or more)
1 piece firm bean cake, 2½ × 2 × 2 inches, cut in small
  ½ inch cubes
Ingredients A:
  1 teaspoon cornstarch
  1 teaspoon Chinese soy bean condiment or substitute
    Japanese *aku miso* (soy bean paste)
  2 teaspoons light soy sauce *(shoyu)*
  1 teaspoon sugar
  ¾ cup chicken broth
  dash MSG (optional)

Mix ingredients A and put aside. Heat skillet or wok. Add oil. Slosh around. Add pork, onions, ginger, garlic and pepper flakes. Toss-fry for 2 minutes until meat is whitish. Add premixed gravy ingredients. Stir-fry until thickened. Add cubed bean cake. Carefully stir. Heat about 2–3 minutes for good flavor harmony. Garnish with a sprinkling of chopped green onion.

Beef with Tomatoes *(Chinese)*

Top of stove   *Serves 4*

With tomatoes available all year round these days one can prepare this favorite dish any time.

1 pound tender beef such as flank, rump, sliced thin ⅛ inch thick
1 medium size onion, cut chunks with 2 inch sides and layers separated
2 green peppers, cut into chunks same size as onions
5 firm tomatoes, skinned and quartered
2 ribs celery, cut diagonally ¼ inch slices
2 Tablespoons oil for frying
Marinate meat in the following:
>   **1 Tablespoon soy sauce *(shoyu)***
>   **1 clove garlic, minced**
>   **1 teaspoon fresh ginger root, grated**
>   **½ teaspoon salt**
>   **1 Tablespoon cornstarch**
>   **1 Tablespoon oil**
Ingredients A:
>   **Mix this in advance in a cup**
>   **½ cup water**
>   **1 Tablespoon cornstarch**
>   **1 teaspoon sugar**
>   **1 teaspoon soy sauce *(shoyu)***
>   **2 Tablespoons sherry wine**
>   **dash MSG (optional)**

Heat skillet or wok on high heat. Add 1 Tablespoon oil. Slosh around. Toss-fry onion, peppers and celery for 2 minutes. Add tomatoes and carefully stir just to heat through so tomatoes will not break up. Takes only about ½ minute. Remove to platter.

Clean skillet. Heat pan and add 1 Tablespoon oil. Add marinated meat. Toss-fry so meat will not stick. While meat is still pinkish add ingredients A and stir until thickened. Add precooked vegetables and carefully toss-fry. Serve with rice or over noodles, either fried or plain boiled.

Heavenly Shrimp Cakes *(Chinese)*

Top of stove   *Serves 4*

A sophisticated way to stretch one pound of shrimp to serve many in a
harmonious blending of ingredients.

   **1 pound shrimp, shelled, deveined, washed, dried well and
     minced fine**
   1 small can water chestnuts, minced fine
   2 large or 3 medium eggs
   3 stalks green onion, minced fine
   1 teaspoon fresh ginger root, grated
   1 Tablespoon sherry wine
   ½ teaspoon salt
   2 Tablespoons cornstarch
   dashes MSG (optional)
   2 Tablespoons oil for frying

Mix all ingredients together except oil. Heat skillet. Add oil. Slosh
around. Scoop large spoonfuls and drop in pan to form patties like
hamburgers. Mixture will tend to be slightly soupy. Fry patties until
lightly browned on both sides. A total cooking time of 5 minutes is all
that will be required. Do not overfry or patties will become dried out.
    Place on a platter lined with shredded lettuce leaves.

   Serve with the following dipping sauce:
      3 Tablespoons rice wine vinegar
      3 teaspoons sugar
      1½ teaspoons fresh ginger root, grated
      dashes of soy sauce *(shoyu)* and MSG (optional)

Your yield with this recipe will be about 12 patties. Now enjoy!

Szechwan Lamb *(Chinese)*

Top of stove *Serves 4*

Lamb is not often thought of as an Oriental meat to be used for every-day but in some areas of China there is much lamb used since it is available. Other meat can be substituted for this recipe easily with good results.

> **1 pound lean lamb, sliced in thin strips from leg**
> **2 Tablespoons oil for frying**
> **Marinade:**
> > **1 clove garlic, minced**
> > **1 teaspoon salt**
> > **2 Tablespoons sherry wine**
> > **1 Tablespoon oil**
> > **2 teaspoons fresh ginger root, grated**
> > **dash MSG**
> > **1 egg, slightly beaten**
> > **1 Tablespoon cornstarch**

Marinate lamb in the above for 1 hour. Heat skillet or wok on high heat. Add oil. Slosh around. Toss-fry lamb slices about 3 minutes. Just enough to be slightly pinkish. Remove and place on hot platter.

> **3 ribs celery, sliced ½ inch wide diagonally**
> **1 cup fresh mushrooms, sliced ¼ inch slices**
> **1 cup edible pod peas, both ends and string removed, left whole unless very long then slice in half diagonally**
> **more oil for frying, if necessary**
> **2 stalks green onions, minced**
> **¾ teaspoon hot chili flakes or substitute several dashes tabasco sauce**
> **Ingredients A:**
> > **2 Tablespoons soy sauce** *(shoyu)*
> > **1½ teaspoons sugar**
> > **1 teaspoon rice wine vinegar**
> > **1 Tablespoon cornstarch**
> > **¼ cup stock**

Clean pan which was used for meat frying. Heat over high heat again. Add a few drops of oil. Slosh around. Toss-fry celery. Add mushrooms and peas tossing for about ½ minute more. Remove to platter. Add sauce ingredients A to pan and cook until thickened. Add all precooked ingredients plus green onions and chili flakes. Heat through about 1 minute. Do not overcook.

Steak Mandarin *(Chinese)*

Broiler or *hibachi*   *Serves 4*

This is an adaptation of Chinese flavors but certainly one which you will appreciate. Be sure to prepare greens with this dish.

1 ½ **pounds flank or other steak, left in one piece**
1 **Tablespoon fresh ginger root, grated**
2 **cloves garlic, minced**
3 **stalks green onions, chopped**
3 **Tablespoons soy sauce** *(shoyu)*
1 ½ **Tablespoons brown sugar**
1 **teaspoon oil**
dashes salt to taste
dashes msg (optional)

Marinate all ingredients together overnight. Turn over once or twice. Light charcoal. When coals are ready and grey ash in color, place steak on rack and broil for about 10 minutes total. Turn over once. This can be prepared in an oven broiler but the flavor is unsurpassed when cooked over coals.

Liver Sweet and Pungent *(Chinese)*

Top of stove   *Serves 4*

A delicate balance is what you should strive for in sweet and sour dishes. Just the right tang countered with proportional sweetness.

> ½ pound chicken livers, cut in half (or substitute beef
>   liver, cut in ¾ inch pieces)
> 1 Tablespoon oil for frying
> 1 clove garlic, minced
> 1 teaspoon fresh ginger root, grated
> ½ teaspoon salt
> dashes pepper and MSG (optional)
> **Sauce ingredients:**
>> 2 Tablespoons cornstarch
>> 1 Tablespoon soy sauce *(shoyu)*
>> ¼ cup vinegar
>> ⅓ cup brown sugar
>> ¾ cup chicken stock
>> dash MSG (optional)

Heat skillet or wok on high heat. Add oil. Slosh around. Add garlic, ginger, liver, salt, pepper and MSG. Toss-fry about 3 minutes until browned and done. Remove to platter. Keep in warm oven while you make sauce.

Mix sauce ingredients and cook in skillet until sauce gets translucent. Prepare the following vegetables and add to sauce cooking about 2 minutes to heat through.

> 1 green pepper, cut into 1 inch square chunks
> 1 medium size carrot, sliced ⅛ inch diagonally and
>   parboiled about 3 minutes and drained
> 2 slices of pineapple, cut in chunks

Pour over cooked liver. Garnish with a few maraschino cherries, if desired.

Festive Moon Salad *(Chinese)*

No cooking   *Serves 4*

This "salad" is adapted from the traditional dish served during the Festival of the Moon. Among the ingredients you will "discover" raw fish is used. Do not let this fact deter you from trying this recipe. You will be amazed that it doesn't taste "raw or strange" at all. I can almost bet that you will "love" this combination.

¾ pound fresh sea bass fillet, sliced into strips about ⅛ × 1 × 1 inch. Squeeze juice of 1 lemon over fish and place in refrigerator (this will make the fish appear "cooked" and the flesh will firm up)

1 Tablespoon peanut oil

Ingredients A:

   ¼ cup preserved Chinese sweet cucumber *(cha gwa)*, slivered

   4 preserved sweet scallions *(rakkyo)*, slivered like matchsticks

   4 stalks green onions, slivered like matchsticks

   8 lettuce leaves, finely shredded

   4 Tablespoons white sesame seeds, toasted

   ½ cup roasted peanuts (no skins), chopped fine

   2 cups deep-fried rice sticks *(mai fun)*, use about ½ cup dry rice sticks as they come from package (refer Chicken Salad recipe page 32)

   1 teaspoon sugar

   ¼ teaspoon dry mustard powder

   ½ teaspoon salt

   ½ teaspoon Chinese 5-spice powder

   2 teaspoons soy sauce *(shoyu)*

   ¼ teaspoon sesame oil

   1 Tablespoon peanut oil

   ½ cup Chinese parsley

Just before serving place lemon marinated fish in a chilled bowl. Add 1 Tablespoon peanut oil. Toss. Add ingredients A and toss lightly. Garnish with ½ cup Chinese parsley sprigs. Be daring and do try this "new" combination of flavors.

Steamed Stuffed Fish *(Chinese)*

Top of stove–steamer *Serves 4*

Simple and yet elegant manner of preparing protein-rich fish.

**1½ pounds bass or trout, left whole, cleaned, washed and
dried off well**
Ingredients A:
½ cup ham, cut like matchsticks
**3 dried black mushrooms, soaked in warm water 15
minutes. Squeeze water out, slice in thin strips**
½ cup bamboo shoots, cut like matchsticks
2 stalks green onions, minced
1 teaspoon fresh ginger root, grated
1 teaspoon salt
dash MSG (optional)
Ingredients B:
2 Tablespoons sherry wine
1 Tablespoon light soy sauce *(shoyu)*
dash sugar
1 Tablespoon oil
salt to taste

Place prepared fish in a heat proof plate like a pyrex pie dish. Stuff
whole fish with ingredients A which have previously been mixed together. Pour ingredients B over stuffed fish.

Get your steamer pot full of boiling water in preparation for steaming. Put the dish of fish on an elevated rack. Cover pan and proceed to
steam for about 20–25 minutes. Make certain that you have free
circulation of steam all around your fish. The fish should be flaky,
tender and moist. Spoon the well flavored juices over the fish and sprinkle some salt just before serving. Garnish with a few sprigs of parsley.

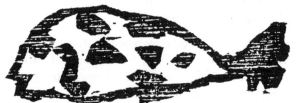

Steamed Celestial Chicken *(Chinese)*

Top of stove–steamer   *Serves 4*

An entirely different sure-fire hit. The fragrance of lemon gives this dish a good change as well as the ever faithful salted black beans *(dau see)* used as a seasoning agent in this recipe.

1 chicken fryer, 3 pounds or larger
Marinade:
    2 Tablespoons salted fermented black beans *(dau see)*,
      washed and drained
    2 cloves garlic, minced
    2 Tablespoons cornstarch
    1½ Tablespoons soy sauce *(shoyu)*
    1 Tablespoon oil
    2 teaspoons sugar
    ½ teaspoon salt
    1 Tablespoon sherry wine
    ½ teaspoon MSG (optional)
    ½ teaspoon sesame oil
    Chinese parsley, chopped
    ½ teaspoon fresh ginger root, grated
    ½ of lemon, squeezed for juice and rind cut into
      quarters

Cut up chicken, bones and all, into chunks 1-inch square. Or, if you prefer, use boneless chicken meat and cut into chunks. Mix all ingredients in a shallow 10 or 11 inch heatproof dish with a high rim. Add chicken pieces and stir well. Prepare steamer full of boiling water. Place dish on rack to steam. Place a dish towel under lid of steamer to prevent droplets of water from falling in dish. Be sure water in lower pan is boiling away for good steam circulation around your chicken dish.

Steam for about 30 minutes. Stir occasionally to distribute flavors and to cook chicken evenly. Adjust flavorings. You may wish to make it a bit sweeter. This goes especially well with hot rice. Remove lemon pieces before serving. Garnish with chopped green onions and Chinese parsley, if desired.

Delectable Clams in Bean Sauce *(Chinese)*

Top of stove   *Serves 4*

This is similar to other seafood dishes but using clams instead. The addition of oyster sauce and hot chili pepper add spice to this gourmet dish.

32 fresh clams with shells, cover clams with salt water ⅓ cup salt to 1 gallon cold water. Let stand 15 minutes. Rinse. Repeat again. Thoroughly wash shells with a brush. Place clams on a rack in a steamer with about 1 cup hot water. Cover the pot tightly and steam for 5 minutes. Remove liquid from clams with care and save in measuring cup

1 ½ Tablespoons light vegetable oil for frying

Ingredients A:

> **2 cloves garlic, smashed, peeled and minced**
>
> **1 Tablespoon fresh ginger root, grated**
>
> **½ teaspoon lemon rind**
>
> **3 Tablespoons fermented salted black beans *(dau see)*, washed, drained in a sieve quickly under the faucet, minced and smashed with flat side of cleaver blade**

Ingredients B:

> **4 Tablespoons sherry wine**
>
> **1 Tablespoon oyster flavored sauce**
>
> **1 teaspoon sugar**
>
> **2 Tablespoons soy sauce**
>
> **½ teaspoon crushed hot chili pepper flakes (optional)**
>
> **1 ½ Tablespoons fresh Chinese parsley (coriander), chopped**
>
> **1½ Tablespoons cornstarch**
>
> **3 Tablespoons water**
>
> **1½ cups broth and clam juice saved from steamed clams**

Heat wok or skillet on high heat. Add oil. Add ingredients A. Toss-fry about 1 minute. Add ingredients B mixed together. Stir. Add steamed clams. Stir constantly while mixture thickens. This should take about 4 minutes on high heat. The sauce coating the shell makes this dish delectable and fantastic feasting.

Serve with plain hot steamed rice. This gravy is a wonderful ambrosia for all gourmets!

Crab with Nappa *(Chinese)*

Top of stove   *Serves 4*

A good blend and balance to give a taste as bright and lively as nature's good greens themselves.

> **1 cup boiling chicken broth**
> **4 cups Chinese cabbage *(nappa)*, cut into 1 inch slices**
> **½ cup water chestnuts, sliced thin**
> **salt to taste**
> **1 Tablespoon oil for frying**
> **3 stalks green onion, chopped**
> **1 teaspoon fresh ginger root, grated**
> **1 clove garlic, minced**
> **1 can crab meat, flaked and all cartilages removed**
> **Ingredients A:**
> > **2 teaspoons cornstarch**
> > **2 Tablespoons water**
> > **2 teaspoons sherry wine**
> > **½ teaspoon sugar**
> > **dash MSG (optional)**

Simmer together broth, *nappa* and water chestnuts for about 5 minutes. Add salt to taste. Put aside. Save broth for use later.

Heat skillet or wok. Add oil and slosh around. Add green onions, ginger and garlic. Toss-fry ½ minute. Add crab meat. Stir about 1 minute. Mix ingredients A and blend with crab mixture. Add reserved broth. Cook until translucent about 2 minutes. Place cooked cabbage and water chestnuts on platter. Put crab mixture over cabbage.

Confetti Noodles *(Chinese)*

Top of stove   *Serves 4*

An entirely unusual treatment for noodles. Actually it is a meal in itself since all kinds of vegetables are combined with the pork to heighten and complement the blandness of the noodles.

> ½ **pound pork with all fat removed, minced**
> 1 **clove garlic, minced**
> 1 **teaspoon fresh ginger root, grated**
> 1 **medium size bamboo shoot, diced (about ¼ cup)**
> ¾ **cup fresh mushrooms, diced**
> 5 **stalks green onions, white portion, shredded for garnish**
>   **and green portion minced for cooking**
> 2 **Tablespoons oil for frying**
> ½ **teaspoon salt**
> ½ **teaspoon sugar**
> 1 **Tablespoon sherry wine**
> ½ **cup stock**
> 1 **Tablespoon soy sauce or** *hoisin* **sauce**
> 2 **Tablespoons brown bean sauce (soy bean condiment),**
>   **crush all beans to make into paste**
> **dash MSG (optional)**

Heat skillet or wok on high heat. Add oil. Slosh around. Add garlic, ginger and pork. Stir-fry about 1½ minutes until pork is whitish in appearance. Add green onions (green portion), bamboo and mushrooms Stir-fry ½ minute. Add balance of ingredients. Stir-fry another 3 minutes to blend flavorings.

> 1 **pound bag fresh egg noodles**
> 1 **cucumber, peeled, cut like matchsticks for garnish**
> **Chinese parsley for garnish, if desired**

Cook noodles in boiling salted water keeping them firm tender. Do not overcook. About 4 minutes or less should be enough cooking time. Drain well and run cold water through noodles. Reheat noodles in a pot of hot water for 1 minute. Drain. Place in 4 large individual bowls. Divide meat sauce and place over hot noodles to one side.

Garnish with white portion of green onions, shredded and cucumbers. Garnishes are meant to be eaten. A sprig or two of Chinese parsley always adds a bit of authentic charm to any dish.

Cornish Game Hen and Vegetables

Top of stove   *Serves 4*

This recipe uses low fat Cornish game hen instead of the usual squab which is most difficult to find if you do not live near a Chinatown ethnic shopping area. And it makes an economical entrée since only one hen is required. Usually in America we feel one hen per person is necessary. This will stretch your budget to feed 4 persons!

**1 Cornish game hen, chopped with cleaver, 1 inch pieces
    bones and all
1 Tablespoon fresh ginger root, grated
1 teaspoon salt
1 clove garlic, minced
1 onion, cut in chunks 1 inch square
1 small eggplant, cut in chunks 1 inch square or 3 Japa-
    nese small type eggplant, sliced
⅓ pound bean sprouts, washed and drained
2 Tablespoons oil for frying
Ingredients A:
    1 teaspoon sesame oil
    2½ Tablespoons brown sugar
    3 Tablespoons soy sauce (shoyu)
    1 teaspoon cornstarch
    dash MSG (optional)
    ½ teaspoon chili flakes (optional)**

Heat skillet on high heat. Add 1 Tablespoon oil. Slosh around. Add ginger, garlic and game hen pieces. Toss-fry and brown until hen is nearly done about 5 minutes. Add onion and eggplant. Toss-fry another 3 minutes or until eggplant is slightly soft. Add ingredients A. Toss-fry until gravy thickens about 3 minutes. Add bean sprouts. Heat through about 1 more minute. Ready to serve.

Beef Congee *(Chinese)*

Top of stove   *Serves many*

Rice prepared in this manner stretches the budget. And at the same time it is most nutritious. Flavoring of *congee* can vary according to one's tastes. There are endless variations. It could be termed a sort of rice soup. And definitely a person could consume 1 cup of this and very little starch would be partaken. *Congee* is called jook by the Chinese.

1 cup raw long grain Patna rice, washed and rinsed
12 cups water
½ teaspoon salt
1½ teaspoons oil
1 pound ground lean beef
½ roll preserved turnip *(chung choi)*, washed carefully,
    drained and chopped fine (approximately ¾ cup)
dash MSG (optional)
Garnishes:
    Chinese parsley, chopped
    green onions, chopped
    fresh ginger root, grated
    sesame oil

Put the rice and water into a deep pot with cover. Add salt and oil. Cover. Bring to boiling point and reduce heat to low. Keep the cover slightly ajar so some steam will escape. Simmer the pot of rice for about 2 or 2½ hours.

Mix the ground beef with the preserved turnip and MSG. Blend in about ⅓ cup water with the meat. Shape beef into about 40 meat balls slightly smaller than a ping-pong ball.

When the rice has cooked the full time put the meat balls into the "rice soup" to simmer about 10 minutes. Taste and add more salt and MSG if desired. When serving use large bowls and a plate filled with the assorted garnishes. People can help themselves. The sesame oil is used much like vanilla is used in a cake recipe. A few drops would be all one would desire in the *congee* serving. A little soy sauce is permissible also. A dash of white pepper makes for zest. A few shreds of raw lettuce make an excellent change in texture to the rice combination.

Sometimes the rice is made without the beef. Raw chicken slices which have been marinated in sauce are dipped into the "rice soup". Occasionally raw fish slices are used. Any combination one could devise would be good.

The Japanese make a very similar rice soup called *okayu*.

Oysters Imperial *(Chinese)*

Top of stove   *Serves 2*

Fresh oysters are available to everyone everywhere in season. So enjoy!

> **1 jar fresh oysters**
> **1 Tablespoon oil for frying**
> **Chinese parsley for garnish**
> **Ingredients A:**
> > **1 teaspoon fresh ginger root, shredded fine**
> > **3 stalks green onion, chopped**
> > **2 teaspoons soy sauce *(shoyu)***
> > **1 teaspoon sherry wine**
> > **dashes sugar and MSG (optional)**

Blanch oysters in hot water to cover for 3 minutes over medium heat. Drain well on paper towels. Heat skillet or wok on high heat. Add oil. Slosh around. Add ginger and oysters. After 1 minute add ingredients A and carefully toss-fry to blend flavors and prevent scorching. Garnish with Chinese parsley.

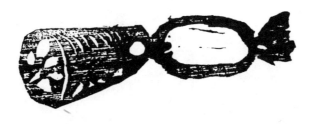

Shrimp and Vegetables *(Chinese)*

Top of stove   *Serves 4*

Here is a hearty combination of shrimp and assorted vegetables. This is another quick to fix food alliance. Soon you will be substituting other vegetables from the ones mentioned in this recipe. Use a free hand and you will probably concoct a masterpiece!

1 pound shrimp, peeled, deveined, washed and cut in half
1 rib celery, sliced diagonally ¼ inch wide
1 medium size onion, halved and sliced ¼ inch wide
1 cup Chinese edible pea pods, ends snipped
½ cup water chestnuts, sliced
6 dried Oriental mushrooms *(shiitake)*, soaked in warm
**   water 15 minutes, squeezed dry and sliced in strips**
2 Tablespoons oil for frying
Ingredients A:
**   1 teaspoon salt**
**   2 teaspoons fresh ginger root, grated**
**   2 Tablespoons light soy sauce *(shoyu)***
**   1 teaspoon sugar**
**   dash MSG (optional)**
Gravy:
**   ½ cup broth mixed with 1 Tablespoon cornstarch**

Marinate shrimp in ingredients A for 15 minutes. Heat skillet or wok on high heat. Add 1 Tablespoon oil. Slosh around. Add marinated shrimp. Toss-fry until pinkish. Add vegetables. Toss-fry 1 minute. Add gravy mixture. Cook until clear and translucent about 1 minute more. Serve with bowls of hot steamed rice.

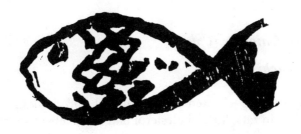

Steamed Fish *(Chinese)*

Top of stove—steamer   *Serves 4*

Variety is the spice of your meals. Here is a nourishing and double quick method of preparing fish. As a bonus you will discover that the fishy odor is not so strong when you steam as when one fries fish. What a relief that is to any cook!

> **1½–2 pounds whole fish, such as sea bass, rock cod, red snapper, scaled and cleaned**
> **Ingredients A:**
> **1 Tablespoon cornstarch**
> **2 Tablespoons soy sauce** *(shoyu)*
> **1 Tablespoon black salted beans** *(dau see)***, washed, drained and mashed**
> **1 Tablespoon** *chung choi* **(salted preserved turnips), washed, drained and chopped fine**
> **1 teaspoon sugar**
> **½ teaspoon salt**
> **1 teaspoon oil**
> **2 Tablespoons fresh ginger root, grated**
> **1 clove garlic, crushed and minced fine**

Place prepared fish heatproof dish. Mix ingredients A in bowl. Rub into fish, both inside and out.

> **2 stalks green onion, shredded fine**

Sprinkle green onions on top. Steam fish for 15–20 minutes until just tender and flaky. Do not overcook. Serve immediately.

Easy, Easy Chicken *(Chinese)*

Broiler or *hibachi* *Serves 3 or 4*

Tender, fresh spring chicken is so healthful and moderately priced. Chicken is low in fats, little cholesterol and an excellent source of protein. Above all chicken is serendipity itself!

> **3 pounds chicken fryer parts, such as legs, thighs or breasts**
> **Marinade:**
> **1 teaspoon dry mustard powder**
> **2 Tablespoons soy sauce *(shoyu)***
> **1 Tablespoon light vegetable oil**
> **2 Tablespoons sesame oil**
> **¾ teaspoon salt**
> **1 Tablespoon cornstarch**
> **2 stalks green onion, chopped**
> **2 Tablespoons Chinese parsley (coriander)**
> **3 or 4 Tablespoons honey**
> **1 teaspoon fresh ginger root, grated**
> **1 clove garlic, minced**
> **dashes pepper and MSG (optional)**

Marinate chicken for at least 2 hours. Turn occasionally. It can be marinated overnight without harm, in fact, it will taste even better. Preheat oven broiler. Broil chicken parts for about 15 minutes on each side. Brush on the chicken any of the left-over marinade during the broiling period. You may wish to use more honey as you broil so that the skin portions will become nicely browned and glazed. Be careful to broil just long enough. Remove from heat while the flesh is still tender and juicy. Not overdone and dry. Chicken is tastiest at this stage.

Desserts

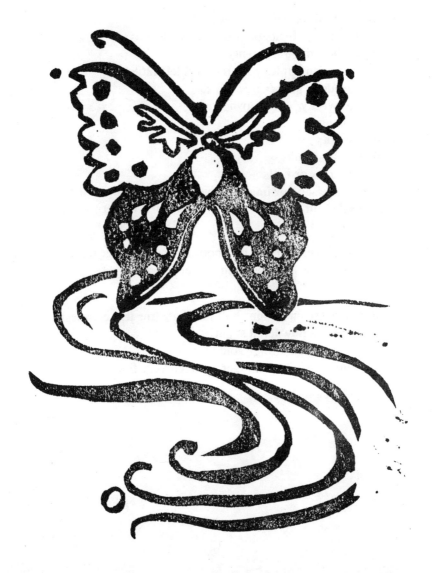

A Dip by Moonlight

No cooking   *Serves many*

Celebrate the end of a magnificent dinner with this light fruit combination with smooth velvety dip. Or serve plain on a bed of crushed
ice for a very sure-fire refreshing hit!

Bamboo skewers such as used for *teriyaki*
Fresh or canned fruits of your choice such as:
   mandarin orange segments
   cubes of crisp apples with red peel left intact
   juicy seedless grapes
   plump sweet whole strawberries
   sliced bananas
   litchee nuts
   pineapple chunks
   melon cubes or balls
   whatever else your imagination or refrigerator conjures up
lemon juice for sprinkling on fruits to prevent browning
   by oxidation

Spear 4 or 5 on each *teriyaki* bamboo skewer. Arrange on a platter with
a dipping bowl near by filled with ginger sauce.
Blend all ingredients together:

2 cups sour cream or sour half and half (for less calories)
5 Tablespoons powdered sugar
1 teaspoon grated orange rind
1 teaspoon crystallized ginger, minced very fine

Savor every luscious bite!

Coconut Dumplings *(Chinese)*

Top of stove *Serves 4*

A delightfully different dessert. Snack in moderation. Too many bitefuls could lead to your weight disaster! These balls will harden up upon being kept over 2 hours so serve them shortly after preparation for "that" special texture–chewy and yet strangely unusual. Delicious!

> ½ **pound** *mochiko* **(sweet glutinous rice flour)**
> **cold water**
> ⅓ **cup sugar**
> **4 Tablespoons crushed roasted peanuts**
> **1 Tablespoon toasted sesame seeds**
> ½ **cup packaged sweetened grated coconut**

Moisten flour with cold water to form a stiff dough. Similar in texture to pie crust. Break into small pieces. Shape balls ¾ inch in diameter. Boil a pot of water and drop dumplings cooking until they come floating to surface. Remove and place in cold water. Combine sugar, peanuts, sesame seeds and coconut on platter. Roll cooled drained lumps in this mixture.

Arrange a few balls on colorful individual plates for dessert.

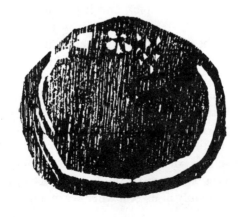

Steamed Chocolate Cake *(Chinese)*

Top of stove–steamer   *Serves many*

Here is an opportunity to have your cake and eat it too—even if you
are watching your weight and calorie intake. Eye appeal may not be
quite inherent here but the flavor is fine. An easy way to make a dessert
in summer without heating up the oven and the house! You could even
make this cake on a camping trip using a wok pan and the same steam
method.

> **4 eggs (room temperature)**
> **⅔ cup sugar**
> **1 teaspoon vanilla**
> **2 Tablespoons cocoa powder, sifted to remove lumps**
> **1 cup flour, sifted**
> **½ teaspoon baking powder**

Beat eggs until very thick. About 5 minutes by hand beater or 2 minutes
by electric beater. Add sugar gradually beating until creamy. Add
vanilla. Sift flour with baking powder and cocoa powder. Fold into egg
mixture. Do not overly mix. Get your steamer pot water boiling at this
point so there will be plenty of steam when you are ready to steam the
cake. Put a sheet of waxed paper on bottom of a 9 inch round pan. No
need to grease pan. Pour batter therein. Place pan on a rack in the
steamer. Cover pot placing a dish towel just under the cover so that the
water drips will not go on the cake. Steam for 20 minutes. Test for
doneness by inserting a toothpick and if it comes out clean then it is
done.

This cake should be allowed to set for a few minutes. Then loosen the
sides and flip over on your hand or rack, quickly remove the paper and
invert cake so that top is upright.

This cake will have a "dull" wet appearance. There will not be the
usual browned crust as if it had been baked. But certainly it matches
other cakes in flavor. There is a certain moistness and rubbery-
sponginess to the texture.

One can garnish "up" or "down" in calories by placing fruit or whip-
ped cream, etc. You will know if today is the day you can splurge or
not. This cake is probably at its best when warm but it is still good when
cold.

An unique method of "baking" a cake!

Fingertip Jewels

No cooking   *Serves many*

This manner of fixing the usual gelatin dessert is quick and easy. The children especially will appreciate this since the gelatin sets very firmly. One can pick and eat with fingers to enjoy the texture. This dessert goes especially well with Asian-style meals I have discovered. And when one serves buffet fashion this is not a messy quick-to-melt delicacy.

3 Tablespoons gelatin or 3 packages unflavored type gelatin
1 cup cold water
2 packages of low calorie flavored gelatin dessert powder
⅓ cup sugar
2 cups hot water

Soften gelatin in cold water. In the meantime mix all other ingredients in a bowl to dissolve. Add softened gelatin and mix well to completely dissolve. Pour in a 9 inch square pan. Refrigerate until set. Cut into diamond shapes or whatever you desire. This is fine for snacks as well as for the ending of a meal. A finger food. Gelatin is most beneficial health-wise since it is protein derived from animal tissues.

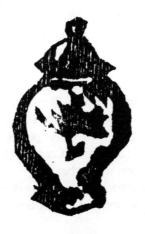

Low Calorie Persimmon Sherbet

No cooking *Serves 6*

You will be free to enjoy your special occasion if you make up this dessert the day before. Serve perhaps a very light thin cooky with this sherbet to bring your memorable dinner to a close.

1 egg, separated
3 Tablespoons sugar
dash salt
1 cup fresh or thawed frozen ripe persimmon pulp, no skin
2 Tablespoons lemon juice
5 Tablespoons ice cold water
5 Tablespoons non-fat dry milk granules

Blend slightly beaten egg yolk, sugar, salt, persimmon pulp and lemon juice. Mix well. Put aside. Beat egg whites slightly in a chilled bowl. Place icy cold water in a cup. Sprinkle dry milk on top. Mix to dissolve. Slowly add to egg white beating all the time. Keep beating until stiff.

Fold in the persimmon mixture. Pour into a large deep ice tray or similar pan. Freeze 3 hours to solid stage. Scoop out or cut into square shape to serve.

Fresh Strawberries

No cooking *Serves many*

A charming manner of serving whole fresh ripe strawberries in season.

Wash and hull, if desired, several baskets of scarlet ripe bruiseless strawberries. Drain on paper towels. Be sure to wash first and then hull after so that the flavor will not be washed away.

Fill a small liqueur glass with sifted powdered sugar, packing well. Place compressed powdered sugar in center of an individual glass plate and surround with luscious whole berries.

If the green hulls have been left on (this is my favorite way) you will discover that they add so much to the decorative touch of this simple dessert.

Glossary

For simplification the Asian names are in italics with (C) and (J) identifying Chinese and Japanese names respectively. The names are necessarily phoenetic and approximate—the ones most commonly used in Western shops.

Agar-agar. *Dai choy gow* (C) or *kanten* (J). Special gelatin derived from seaweed used generally for desserts although other applications exist. Sold in noodle-like strips or in long cube-shape crinkly blocks.

Age (J). Deep-fried soy bean cake. Brown, crispy surface. Inside at times almost hollow.

Bamboo shoots. Ivory colored crunchy shoots of large bamboo canes usually only canned ones available in Western countries. Occasionally fresh ones to be had in Chinatown shops in season.

Bean cake. *Dow foo* (C) or *tofu* (J). Nutritious protein rich custard-like squares of coagulated soy bean purée. Bland flavor.

Bean sprouts. Mung bean sprouts are very white, highly nutritive and can be utilized in many ways either raw or cooked.

Bean threads. *Sai fun* (C). Wiry dried thin translucent noodles prepared from mung beans. Soak in hot water before use for about 20 minutes. Also called cellophane noodles, silver noodles and long rice. A good substitute for Japanese *ito-gonyaku* or *shirataki*. Cooked in combination with meats and vegetables or in soups and salads.

Black fermented salted beans. *Dau see* (C). Strong pungent flavor. Keeps indefinitely. Firm to touch but beans can be crushed between fingers. Packed in plastic bags. Authentic Chinese seasoning agent. Odor comes basically from bits of dried fish mixed with salted beans and definitely has no substitute.

Brown bean sauce. *Mein see jeong* (C). Chinese soy bean condiment. A very salty brown mixture of yellow soy beans, flour and salt which adds a special flavor to cooked dishes.

Chinese cabbage or celery cabbage. *Nappa* (J). Crinkled pale green leaves with pure white stems. Generally tightly compacted heads. Used raw or cooked. Excellent adapted to Western dishes. Not potent like regular cabbage since it is more of the celery-type family.

Chinese chard. *Bok choy* (C). Milky white stalks with dark green leaves. Looks like Swiss chard but milder in flavor.

Chinese parsley. *Yuen sai* (C). This fresh coriander is an authentic seasoning and flavor found in Chinese cooking. Do not substitute regular parsley. Easily grown at home with coriander seeds—be sure to buy non-treated type seeds at the grocery shops. *Cilantro* is the Mexican name for coriander.

Daikon (J). Japanese white long radish. Often used raw and puréed. Very excellent enzymes in *daikon* which help digestion of starches in particular. Can be cooked like turnips. Sometimes *daikon* is referred to as the "workhorse" of Japanese cuisine!

Dashi (J). Japanese seaweed and fish soup base.

Dried mushrooms. *Doong goo* (C) or *shiitake* (J). Thick black mushrooms which are quite expensive but a little goes a long way in yielding a woodsy flavor. Soak in warm water for 15–20 minutes before use. Save water for cooking being careful not to use sediment that may have accumulated at bottom.

Edible chrysanthemum leaves. *Shungiku* (J). Generally sold in bunches and used by both the Chinese and the Japanese in their cuisine. Plant is garland chrysanthemum.

Five-spice powder. *Ng heung fun* (C). A Chinese fragrant mixture of star anise, Chinese pepper, fennel, cloves and cinnamon. Try even using it for Western cooking such as for cookies—a delightful surprise.

Ginger. Bulbous light brown root with special zip. Do not use dried powdered ginger as a substitute. Leave out of recipe if unavailable although fresh ginger root along with garlic are the inseparable companions of genuine Chinese cookery.

Gobo (J). Burdock. Long brown thin roots with white flesh. Used in much the same way as carrots.

Gyoza skins (J). Round noodle paste skins, fresh or frozen. Many uses: traditional or imaginative. Some of my students use these skins for Italian raviolis!

Hoisin sauce (C). A soybean sauce flavored with garlic and chili.

Lop cheong (C). A very flavorful spicy pork sausage which keeps a long time in refrigerator or can be frozen.

Lotus root   *Renkon* (J).Fresh roots look like huge sausages linked together. Brown skin but with pearly white lacy-look when sliced crosswise.

MSG. Monosodium glutamate. A natural seasoning derivative that enhances hidden flavors in foods. Prepared from wheat, sugar beets and other natural plant sources. Use in moderation.

Mirin (J). Sweet rice wine. Wine made from glutinous sweet rice with sugar added. Used for cooking Japanese foods in particular. Sherry wine with a bit of sugar added could be a substitute.

Miso (J). Soy bean paste. Japanese type used in soups, salads and for cooking. Made from soy beans, malt and salt. Several different "strengths". *Shiro miso* is mildest and my recommendation to Westerners for a starter. *Aka miso* is very pungent and takes a period of getting used to the taste—very salty and strongly flavored.

Mochiko (J). See sweet glutinous rice flour.

Mung bean sprouts. See bean sprouts.

Nama yaki dofu (J). Fried firm soy bean cake (not *age*).

Oyster flavored sauce. Made from oysters, soy and brine. Gives a distinctive touch to Chinese dishes.

Preserved sweet cucumbers. *cha gwa* (C). Sweet and syrupy slices of small pickled cucumbers. Very crunchy and can be served plain as pickles, in salads or as garnish. Either in jars or in tins.

Preserved turnips. *chung choi* (C). A moist salt pickled turnip. Rinse well under water faucet before use to remove excess salt. Some turnips come rolled like golf balls and others are long and slender.

Rakkyo (J). Pickled sweet scallions with only the bulb portion used. Use for addition to sweet and sour dishes or plain as appetizers.

Red bean curd. *Nam yoi* (C). Fermented bean curd squares with liquor and aromatic spices. Crush before using. Truly an Oriental cheese!

Rice. Patna or long grain used for Chinese cooking generally cooked to this proportion: 1 cup rice to 1¼ cups water. Cooked rice is loose and flaky grained.

Medium grain used for Japanese cooking generally cooked to this proportion: 1 cup rice to 1 cup water. Important that this rice type be well washed before use to remove polish. Sticky and cooked grains hold together nicely.

Rice sticks. *Mai fun* (C). Rice flour used to form opaque wire like strings. Similar to bean threads but different texture when cooked. Can be deep-fried for use in dishes such as chicken salad in which case do not soak before use—use dry when dropping into hot oil.

Rice wine vinegar. *Chit chu* (C) or *su* (J). Mild vinegar made from sweet glutinous rice.

Sake (J). Japanese rice wine. Sherry makes adequate substitute for cooking.

Seaweed. *Konbu* (J). Very tough, dark green thick sheets of tangle seaweed used basically for making broth.
Nori (J). Laver seaweed prepared in rectangular sheer sheets.
Wakame (J). Delicate seaweed often used for salads and soups.

Sesame oil. A fragrant reddish brown oil with distinctive sesame flavor. Use sparingly a few drops at a time for subtle taste in foods.

Shichimi **pepper** (J). *Togarashi* (J). Japanese 7-spices. A mixture of many spices giving a "zip" to foods. Basically Japanese red pepper, sesame seeds, orange peel, seaweed, chili and other spices.

Shirataki (J). Japanese yam noodles. Almost like long strips of rubber bands and used most often for *sukiyaki*-type dishes.

Soy sauce. *See yow* (C) or *shoyu* (J). A salty sauce from soy beans, wheat and salt. Japanese all purpose *shoyu* is best for both cooking and table use. *Shoyu* used exclusively for testing of these recipes.

Soy bean sprouts. Pea sprouts. Young white sprouts of soy beans. Sprouts have large beans attached which are crunchy and most nutritious.

Sukiyaki **meat.** Tender thinly sliced beef rib eye or fillet meat.

Togarashi (J). See *shichimi* pepper.

Wasabi (J). A green colored sharp flavored horseradish sold in dried powdered form to be mixed with water to form a "hot" paste.

Water chestnuts. Brown fuzzy bulb looking vegetable when peeled it is very white inside. Fresh ones are most delicate, sweet and crunchy. Canned ones are more commonly available in Western shops.

Index

Shabu-Shabu, 40
Shrimp and Vegetables, 78
Soy Bean Sprouts with Pork, 60
Spanish Mackerel with Ginger, 56
Special Turkey, 35
Spinach Relish, 16
Steak Mandarin, 67
Steamed Celestial Chicken, 71
Steamed Chocolate Cake, 84

Steamed Fish, 79
Steamed Stuffed Fish, 70
Stuffed Cucumber, 61
Szechwan Lamb, 66

Tofu Teriyaki Bites, 31

Yakitori, 45

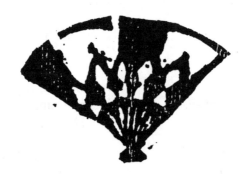